So This Is Nursing

Milicent McCalla

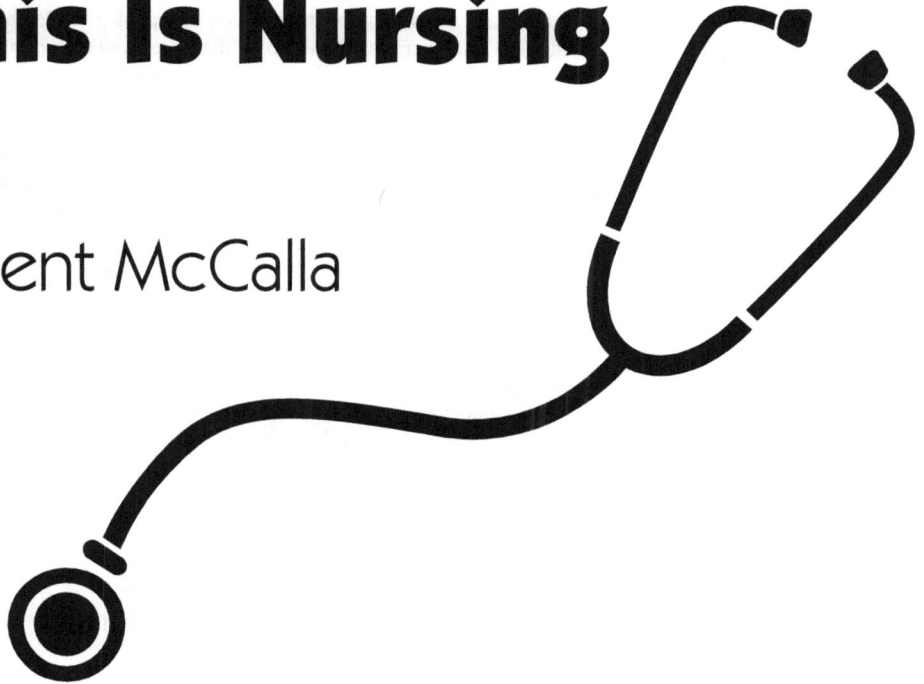

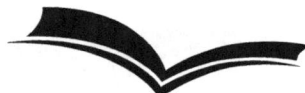

TEACH Services, Inc.
PUBLISHING
www.TEACHServices.com • (800) 367-1844

Copyright © 2013 TEACH Services, Inc.
ISBN-13: 978-1-57258-930-8 (Paperback)
ISBN-13: 978-1-57258-931-5 (ePub)
ISBN-13: 978-1-57258-932-2 (Kindle / Mobi)
Library of Congress Control Number: 2012956075

Published by

TEACH Services, Inc.
PUBLISHING
www.TEACHServices.com • (800) 367-1844

Table of Contents

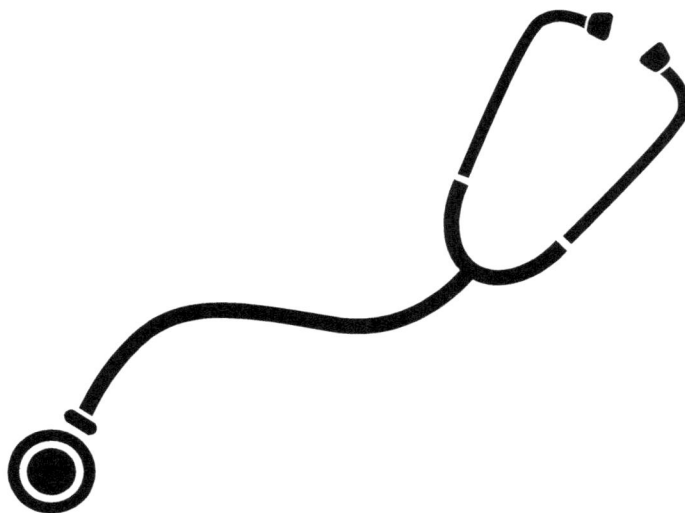

Chapter One

My First Hospital Visit

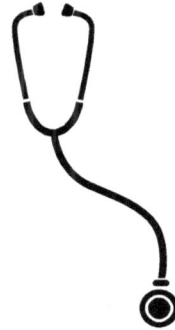

Hospitals are places designed to mend bodies and minds, but they can become environments in which imaginations and emotions run rampant. They are not always people friendly and can at times be compared to the halls of justice where not everyone gets what he or she bargains for. An uncomplicated birth of a child or the miraculous recovery of one whose illness seemed near hopeless are significant moments to dance and sing about.

On other occasions, the very thought of losing a loved one to death can be mind-boggling, striking fear and dread in the hearts of family and friends. "Why is there so much suffering? Why is life so unfair?" we are prone to ask at times. The answers oftentimes don't make sense but in the meantime, we must keep some measure of hope alive in order to go on. Life can be a very bitter *pill* to swallow.

I have a library of memories I have been collecting and saving over the years, and it all started when I was a youngster. It took one visit to a hospital and my fate was sealed. The memory of that visit is as vivid today as it was when it happened. I was just about five years old—a big intelligent five year old. I came face to face with the brutal reality of how fragile life really is, and I did not like it one bit!

What necessitated the hospital visit was that my dad, who at that point in my life was as strong as Leo the lion, was sick and in the hospital. My dad was the rock on which my siblings and I found refuge, stability, and safety. Nothing could go wrong when he was with us. At times I even thought he was God! After all, isn't God supposed to love, protect, guide, and look out for us when we cannot fend for ourselves? I thought my problems would always be small ones and he would always be there to solve them for me. When I placed my little hand in his big hand, I felt safe and secure.

But when my dad became quite ill, I felt betrayed. Upon arriving at the hospital, I found him in a hospital bed wrapped up in yards of bandages just like an Egyptian mummy. He had a needle poked into his arm with some type of "water" running into it. I tried to figure out where the "water" was going. Was it draining out into his bed? It was like a leaking tap: *drip, drip, drip*! As far as I was concerned, water was for cooking, washing, bathing, and drinking. It was not supposed to be going where it was going! Little did I realize that what Papa was actually receiving was indeed a drip, or intravenous fluid!

Cuts and bruises covered his body. This was not supposed to be happening. He had promised us, his children, that he would always be there for us no matter what, and there he lay, defenseless, with one step between him and death. I was not amused; in fact, I was quite annoyed, but at the same time, I was hopeful he would somehow solve the problem as he always did.

My dad had been involved in a serious motor vehicle accident and had sustained some very life-threatening injuries. Eyewitness accounts and then later his own account of what had happened on that fateful night of the accident convinced me that only Divine providence snatched him from the very jaws of death. My dad was hit by a car, which pinned him against a concrete column of a bridge. The column gave way because of the impact and he fell several feet down the side of that bridge. He fractured several ribs and coughed up frank blood for a while, but he defied death, which he later repeated several times during the course of his long life.

After the accident he hovered between consciousness and a "twilight state" as he described it. He heard voices but was unable to respond. In his twilight state, he oftentimes repeated concern for his family. "God, I am not ready to go. Who will take care of my children and my wife? They need me. I cannot leave them, not yet, Lord, not yet!" When he was tap-dancing between life and death, his family was his greatest concern.

I was born with a streak of nosiness as well as curiosity. Nicely put, I was *intrusively inquisitive*—I definitely had an inquiring mind. My siblings and I were not quite prepared for that moment in the hospital. The place smelled of strong medicine, pungent disinfectant, sickness, and death. It was clearly a place where most people would rather not be. But I didn't want to be any place else because, you see, the most important person to me in the whole wide world was there!

Papa was a man who did not hesitate to spar with us, give us piggyback rides, and hand wrestle with us, sometimes letting us win just to teach us valuable object lessons. He taught us that in the future we would make mistakes and mess up at times, but we should have the will and determination to pick up the pieces and start all over again.

As we looked at this great man lying on the bed, for once in our young lives, we were afraid to approach him or even touch him. That gave me an unnerving feeling. We were not equipped to deal with such stressors at that stage of our lives.

We stood at a safe, comfortable distance from Papa's bedside. The tension in the room was dense. Someone had to break it, but who would do so? As the intrusively inquisitive one, I decided I had to break the ice. I went up to Papa like a trouper with my heart in overdrive and a grin from ear to ear. What the dickens was I grinning about? Fear gripped my very soul! I was just putting on a brave front, thus making it easier for everyone else.

I approached with caution. What if I touched him and caused him pain? What should I say to him? Some of my earliest recollections were those of hearing Papa quoting some philosophical statement that sounded a bit advanced for me, or even for him, but somehow they made me stop and think. He would say stuff like, "See yourself there." "Act as if…" "Reach for the stars…" "Nothing is impossible when you put your trust in God." "A great man shows his greatness by the way he treats the little man." Well I decided to try out one of those statements in this state of emergency, so I acted as if … I was a *nurse* in my own right, and the rest is history!

I touched Papa's chest bandages ever so gently and began to do my own "physical assessment" of him and of the situation. Then I fired off a series of questions. "So how are you feeling? Are you having any pain? Did you eat? What is that thing in your arm? Are the nurses taking good care of you? Did you sleep well during the night? When are you coming home?"

I observed his skin and touched his brow. He didn't feel hot, so I knew he didn't have a fever. His chest rose and fell, so I was quite sure he had respirations. He could raise his arms and lift his legs; therefore, I told myself he was not paralyzed. There was no obvious neurological deficit, so I deduced that he would soon be walking home!

The questions kept flying out of my mouth as fast as my tongue and brain could tailor them! I didn't really expect answers. I only needed to talk to him and to realize that he could talk back to me; nothing else really mattered. My "physical assessment" confirmed that he was orientated to time, place and person! I then upgraded his condition from critical to stable! The tension finally abated and all exhaled in unison. The prognosis seemed good. A nurse, a little shy of a nurse practitioner or doctor, to boot, was born at that moment! Papa was going to be alright and speedily, as well.

Time, which had stood still for all of us, began to flow as it usually did. Time and timing can be worlds apart, but I had a perfect timing that day and that has been one of the classic collections in my library of memories. A beautiful nurse then entered the room and came by my dad's bedside. She made small talk with us and with Papa, and then she gently placed her hand on my head and smiled at me. I swore I was touched by an angel! To me she was an angel minus wings, halo, and harp! I told her with childlike innocence, "I am going to be a nurse just like you."

She then said these words, which have been my guiding light for decades, "You can become anything you wish as long as you study hard and keep your wishes alive."

Those words sent shivers down my spine. I saw myself there. Papa's philosophy, coupled with that nurse's endorsement, were enough to trigger my choice of profession, the most noble and rewarding calling that we, the unsung heroes and heroines, over the years and over the world have come to embrace and love.

I never got another chance to see my "angel" in human form again, but over the years I have thought about her, and even now when the going gets tough, I can still hear her words ringing in my ears. I wish I could have met her again, just to say thanks for playing a part in what I have become. One might never know how far one's influence might go, so one needs at all times to leave a good impression. Her uniform, shoes, cap, and stockings were immaculately clean and white. I saw myself garbed in like fashion. After more than three decades, I am still wearing my white uniform, which has become my trademark. Papa was my first patient. I never received a penny, but the experience, time, and effort were worth far more than money or praise.

Chapter Two

Elementary School Days

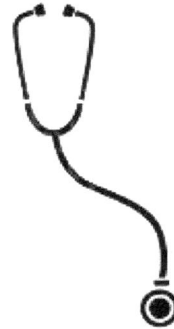

Elementary school, some four miles from home, was the first port of call on my educational voyage. It was a long, choppy, sometimes rough passage, but with the support of kinfolks and the unfailing love and care of God, I weathered the storms and reached my desired haven. It is said that the farther one goes down the mountainside, the clearer one remembers things that were at the top. I can subscribe to that, because events that happened many years ago still remain quite clear to me. I still remember my first grade teacher, how she walked and talked and the way she smelled, no expensive perfumes or lotions, just an honest to goodness clean homemade fragrance. Teachers in those bygone days were considered by most of us to be infallible. The sun rose and set on them.

My mother was my first teacher and continued thus even unto high school. I give a lot of credit to her for her input, but in the wider sphere of learning, my first grade teacher, heaven bless her, fine-tuned what my mom began in a structured classroom environment. Most everyone should be able to identify with this. Can you remember the first day or even the first week away from home when you entered a classroom with a whole bunch of strangers? If you were as bashful as I was, then you would remember the sweaty palms and rapid heartbeat. School was not my favorite spot—it was stressful!

My teacher made us identify who we were within the first moments she laid eyes on us. It was roll call time. Now in the neck of the woods where I grew up, we were called every name except the one that was legally ours on our birth certificates. We were given "pet names." As far as I was concerned, my name was "Joy" because that was what my family and friends called me. When I was asked my name for the first time outside of my family circle, of course, I answered, "My name is Joy McCalla." I was duly informed by my teacher, much to my embarrassment and to the amusement of my classmates, that no child by that name was present in her classroom.

"Child, do you not know your own name?" she asked.

That question gave the kids in my class weapons to destroy my ego. I had to think fast to redeem myself.

"They call me 'Joy,' but my real name is Millicent McCalla, Teacher."

"Okay, young lady, from now on, remember to use that name here! You are not at your home."

What a professional snob! From that point onward, I did not care what the other kids thought because I convinced myself that my teacher was not human. Those folks who used chalk to write on blackboards were not earthlings at all! Then on other days I sort of psyched myself into believing that she might have had a "pet name" as well so she could have related to my predicament. Then I asked myself, Who am I kidding?

But the dust settled, and I adjusted to the routine of going to school some four miles away. You might be wondering why I keep repeating the distance to and from school. I was not walking or running that long distance twice daily to keep in shape or for the health benefits I learned about later in school. I had no choice. I could not by any stretch of my imagination come up with an excuse for being absent or late to school. The distance, the chores that had to be done prior to leaving home, the rain and heat—nothing was worth mentioning. Some days the sun's rays would be so fierce and brutal that a nice refreshing shower and a long glass of ice-cold lemonade would have been a welcome treat for me and all the other long-distance runners, when we finally reached school.

But there was no time to daydream or have flights of fancy! School was a very serious business. With the limited time that was given to each child by our country's government to get a free education up until about age fifteen, the future rested to a great extent squarely on each child's shoulders. We were given the same hours, relatively the same curriculum and the same opportunities to acquire tools to function in the future. Some grabbed the fundamentals and made great success stories for themselves while others chose the easier way out. They wasted time and ended up being liabilities.

Fortunately, school wasn't all bad. In fact, I loved writing class where I could use my imagination. I remember one such writing assignment. I really believe the exercise was geared to give my teacher some idea of what her pupils would eventually become in the future. I believe that she thought that someday, some far off day, she would look back with pride and savor even one of her pupils' success stories. My classmates and I had to write from our hearts a paper titled "When I grow up." I decided to give it my best shot. But how far into the future could a seven-year-old child look? My dad's "Act as if ..." statement and the nameless nurse's endorsement gave me my first sentence. Little did I then realize that the white, blank page on which I wrote that composition would one day give me the courage to honestly write this book from my heart. My pencil approached my blank piece of paper with fear and trembling, but as words began to appear, I felt as if I was being transformed into a real author.

"When I grow up, I am going to be a good nurse. I want to help sick people get better. I will give them pills and injections. I will care for them and love them. I will wear pretty white uniforms."

If I had the courage then as I have now, I would have added a resounding "Amen." I remember misspelling injection. After all, that was quite a big word for an amateur first-time autobiographer. I am sure I mentioned a few more fancy things, but I am unable to quote them now, but I am quite certain my teacher got the message!

I never second-guessed my intended profession. I put all my eggs in one basket and was determined to guard that basket viciously day and night. As I grew older and began to study human behavior, I learned that most people need to have alternatives in order to deal with possible failures or losses. In other words, they should have a Plan B. I never had another plan that involved any other letter in the alphabet! I knew exactly what I wanted at age five, and I never explored any other career choices. Through the years, I have had moments when I thought of saying to the powers that be, "I have had enough; I am not coming back," but my first love, nursing, keeps me going in spite of the odds. I mentioned in my composition, "I am going to be a good nurse," not "I think I might become a good nurse." Good is a relative term, but every day I endeavor to become a better nurse than I was the shift before. There is always room for improvement.

My thoughts in my essay were next scrutinized by my teacher. In those bygone days, I observed that teachers were very generous with the use of their red ink pens. They would strike through a misspelled word like a guillotine, underline, and make big comments, and they seemed to get an enormous kick out of doing so. To a nervous inexperienced child, red ink meant warfare, red ink meant danger! I earned my first red ink mark when I ventured into the unknown territories of big words and misspelled injection. I watched my teacher attentively as she used her red ink pen, and from her facial expressions, I knew she was not too impressed with what was written by my classmates and maybe, by me as well.

Why should she be so mad? I thought. Writing was something new and strange to all of us. We were just rookies sent out on our first beat. Heaven help us! After what seemed like eternity for her to finish reading our compositions, the moment of truth came. She stepped out from behind her desk, which I believed was her throne, and came and stood over me.

"What is your name again, little girl?"

God must have dispatched His fastest angel to loosen my tongue and give me clarity of speech. He knew my fragile little ego could not take a second assault in less than a week of my school life!

"My name is Milicent May McCalla, teacher." I made sure I gave her my full name. I was just about to add my date of birth and mailing address, but I deferred that data! She would have considered me fresh and cheeky!

"Very good," she said.

Fear, coupled with her "very good" comment, caused beads of perspiration to issue from pores in my body that I never knew existed. My teacher smiled at me, but I wondered about the motive behind the smile. Was I becoming a bit paranoid at my young age? Her smile reminded me of the smirk my dog, Rover, would have made, exposing his fangs before he chased our neighbors' chickens from our property, threatening to devour them alive! I soon discovered, however, that her smile was genuine. That smile was like a benediction.

"Little girl, do you really mean what you just wrote?" my teacher asked.

"Yes, teacher," I replied.

"Well, never forget it because I am sure that one day you will be a fine nurse."

That was music to my ears. I was transported to the seventh heaven on wings of humble pride. My soon-to-hit-the-bestsellers'-list essay was taken to a teacher next door. It was as if I had struck gold. I saw my teacher with her colleague standing at the doorway pointing a finger in my direction. Then they both waved to me as if I were Queen Elizabeth of England! I could not wait for lunch to tell my siblings of my good fortune.

By the following day, however, my good fortune spiraled downward sharply like a bad day at the New York Stock Exchange! I was heading for a recession! You see, I could write legibly and nicely by printing in bold letters, but I had no idea how to write in cursive form. I had observed my mother over the years writing beautifully in flowing style. She joined one letter to the next with ease and precision. I needed to impress my teacher so badly that I *knew* what I was doing so I thought of a quick fix to the problem. I solicited the help of my big sister. After all, isn't that what big sisters are for? When lunch came, I went to my sister and told her of my impending doom if I could not write in cursive by the time I chopped and swallowed my lunch and returned to class. Time was of the essence; there was not one second to lose! I rough copied the assignment in bold letters as I was accustomed to writing and asked my sister to show me how to transform it into my teacher's expectation.

Yvette, my sister, came up with the ultimate readymade solution. Why not do the whole thing herself and get it over with? Who would know the difference anyway? Boy, were we in for an enormous surprise! I began to chew my lunch as a human being ought because I had everything under control and a bit of time to kill as well.

Classes resumed at last for the second part of the day. I remember clearly that our times table was drilled into our brains from the very beginning of our school life. We had no calculators then so we had to memorize our times table. "Two ones two, two twos four, two threes six, two fours eight…" Once our little mental exercise was completed, it was time to hand in our assignment in cursive!

I handed my script in to my teacher with a sinking feeling that I was soon to be discovered. The thing I greatly feared was quickly realized. It is said that the road to hell is paved with good intentions. Little did my sister and I realize that my teacher was very much familiar with Yvette's penmanship because Yvette had been a student of hers just two years before!

The moment of reckoning finally came. My teacher came and stood over me. I did not particularly like that position, but I thought that since I had been singled out as the next Florence Nightingale just a few hours before I was still in good standing with her. I was wrong. Her whole demeanor changed. She did not view me walking through the corridors of time administering medications, including injections, and saving lives. She saw me as a fraud, a phony, and a cheat, to say the least.

"Is this your handwriting, child?" she asked. My name was quickly forgotten.

"Yes, teacher, I wrote it during lunch break."

"Are you sure that this is your handwriting, child?"

"Yes, teacher," I replied.

"I am going to show you that this is not your handwriting because I still have with me a book with your sister's handwriting in it," she replied.

She produced the book and a leather strap. She hit me across my back, which felt like the sting from the cat-o'-nine-tails! My dad, who was once a soldier in the first battalion of the Jamaican Regiment, informed us that if we played the fool we would feel the sting of the cat-o'- nine-tails, a knotted rope reserved for flogging unruly folks in the military.

Because of my poor choices, I was flogged publicly for the first time, to my shame, and I have never forgotten such indignity. Back then teachers had license to punish students a little short of the death sentence. Their only concern was to make sure their students' eyeballs were left intact! Then she had the nerve to preach to me in my agony. Maybe she wanted to console my soul, but all I felt was more humiliation. "Speak the truth and speak it ever, cost it what it will. He who hides the wrong he did, does the wrong thing still!"

I felt like a fool, but I was determined to repair the damage. I purposed in my heart I would atone for the sin of lying. If I had to pay dearly for lying because of the gravity of the situation, then I thought to myself that grown persons—including adults and heads of state who told "white lies" or called it "executive privilege"—should be punished because they should know better. Wishful thinking, indeed! After all, it wasn't my fault I didn't know what I was doing at that point in my scholastic pursuit!

I arrived at home in a down mood; I looked much the same way I had observed my beloved dog, Rover, looking when he was troubled. He would hold his head down and put his tail between his hind legs. But my melancholy feeling didn't last long. I soon rebounded thanks to my mother offering me a crash course in cursive. "Miss I," as she is affectionately called by everyone, was my own private tutor. She patiently showed me how this style of writing was done. Later I thought to myself, *Wow, this is ridiculously easy after all!* I never thought I could become a pro so quickly! I returned to school the next day ready and waiting to show off my beautiful penmanship.

My mother quoted another philosophical idea to me from Shakespeare's *Hamlet*,

"This above all: to thy own self be true,

And it must follow, as the night the day,

Thou canst not then be false to any man."

I swear my mom was in love with William Shakespeare, for she quoted him often over the years! My dad then put in his two cents worth of admonitions. "Honesty is the best policy, and lying lips are an abomination to the Lord but they that deal truly are His delight."

Can you imagine a seven year old being told quotes with five-syllable words like abomination to her? What on earth were those quotations supposed to mean? Were they nuts? Years later I got the full significance of those witty phrases and quotations and have been applying them for most of my life except when "discretion is the better part of valor" and when "not all truths need to be known." My favorite is from William Blake's "Auguries of Innocence":

"A truth that's told with bad intent

Beats all the lies you can invent."

My teacher was perplexed as to how quickly I had mastered the art of writing. I never revealed my source. I thought the punishment meted out the previous day didn't quite fit the crime, so I decided then and there to dislike school intensely. I could not wait to finish and get out, but dropping out was never an option. My parents would have literally killed me. My dad told me that as a soldier he had been taught the easiest and quickest way to kill an enemy. He would have gladly substituted enemy for child, and believe me, I loved my life!

I think it's okay to have a little dread of your parents. But all kidding aside, I knew that my dad loved us dearly, but as his kids, we knew we were not pals, he was our father! He was the final authority in the house. Parents make decisions for us until we are free to make our own decisions—good or stupid. Our parents save us from many a pitfall and danger that we never quite realized existed.

I have no shortage of memories of my growing-up years from elementary school through high school and beyond. Some were happy ones that I "framed" and kept on my memory wall, while others I consciously shut out or deleted as I tried to cope with life.

I believe that elementary school creates the fundamentals of education in a child's academic life. If that base is firm and if only the best materials are given and used, chances are that there is no limit to what that person can become. All the ingredients needed to articulate the English language and grammar and other subjects I received from my elementary school education. High school then put on the finishing touches.

Because I grew up with older siblings around, I remember being introduced to textbooks such as "First Aid in English," "Students' Companion," and "Looking at Life" from the word go. "Looking at Life" was a bit advanced for me at that time because it was a high school biology textbook. But you should be aware by now that I was quite nosy! Those textbooks gave me a head start. Even though English is my native tongue, I had to learn English! I wanted to know why I spoke the way I did, not just because of tradition but by reason. Strange, isn't it? I tip my hat and raise my glass to my teachers back then. Heaven bless them. Many have passed away, but their wisdom and memories are alive and well.

As I previously mentioned, at that time, education was free. All we had to do was show up in the appropriate attire and be on time. I remember my blue and white uniform, white socks, and black shoes. The boys were smartly garbed in their starched khaki uniforms with seams so sharp as if they could cut on contact! The girls took great pride in wearing the whitest blouses and nicely pressed pleated skirts. We never had a lot of uniforms, but we always appeared clean and neat.

We didn't have metal detectors then because guns and knives were not included in our school bags. Not many school bags existed either! A few stones were flung here and there as if we were living some place in the Middle East and fistfights were not uncommon, but no permanent injuries or damages resulted from putting a fist in someone's jaw when he or she felt disrespected or if the adversary needed to be chastised! When those scenes were over, it was back to the business of being schoolmates. I showed up at school daily, but if the truth be known, school in all its levels was never my favorite place, so I could not wait to get out, close the books, and grab life by the horns.

Of course, if we are honest with ourselves, how many of us really loved school? Most of us could not wait for weekends, vacation time, rain, snow days, or even the threat of a category five hurricane to hit land so that we would not have to go to school! We could not wait for recess and lunchtime so that we could have a break during the school day. When my elementary school days were over, I knew I was one step closer to my dream and doing what I really wanted to do. Instead of going to school, I wanted to work as a nurse.

In those days, it was unusual for principals to communicate one on one with students. Mine was different. I never associated principals as being a part of the general population. They were the bigwigs of society. It was only as I got older and, I guess wiser, that I realized that they were prone to goofing up as badly as the rest of us and sometimes even bigger. My principal, Mr. Cleveland Kean, who was one of my mother's schoolmates, gave to me a mandate and his blessings upon leaving elementary school, and there was no way I could ever disappoint him.

There was a Jamaican singer who gained international fame by the name of Millie Smalls. My principal usually called me Millie Smalls after that famous singer. Just before leaving for high school, he called me into his office and gave me a parting gift. It was not wrapped, and it could not be held or touched, but the value outweighed any package put together. He gave me a simple truth that I have put into practice ever since.

He said, "Millie, I wish that you would become a teacher just like I, but I know what you want, and nobody can stop you. Make me a promise. Promise me that you will study hard, focus on what's important, and always follow your dreams."

That promise was not hard to keep. Many years later I had the distinct pleasure of having him as a guest at my parents' golden anniversary celebration and introducing him to the audience. He was totally unprepared for that moment. I actually reminded him of the boost he gave to me many years before. It was then payback time.

Chapter Three

My High School Years

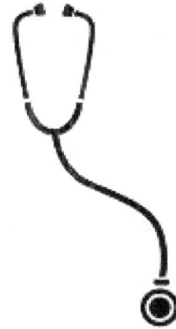

I was blessed with parents who possessed insight, vision, and *uncommon sense*. We often hear folks talk about using common sense to solve problems as if that skill is readily available to everyone. If it were so common, how come so many people lack perceptiveness? My folks' "uncommon sense" was hinged on their dependence on God, willingness to change the norm of the little tight community in which we lived, and ability to act and think independently.

My parents, with their limited resources, thought that by giving us a private high school Christian education we, as their children, would be ambitious enough to take it from there and aspire to be the best we were capable of becoming. From my earliest recollection, they coined this phrase, "Our God-given responsibility," which they exercised as if it were a badge of honor. Their "God-given responsibility" was a self-imposed mandate, and it was not negotiable. All my worldly possessions were stuffed into one brown suitcase, and I was *sent* to a high school in Port Antonio in the parish of Portland, which was outside of my hometown. I didn't have any other choice. I was practically on my own, but I had no dread because the confidence my parents placed in me and the trust I had in God were quite sufficient to sustain me.

I am not a religious fanatic, but I firmly believe in a God who does things in His own time and in His own way and that human beings are powerless to alter His plan no matter how hard they try. But He also gives us choices! When He gives dreams and insight, He also provides the means by which those dreams can be realized. He is Jehovah-jireh, the God who always provides, and the God who always sees to it! He sometimes uses people, just ordinary people, to be there at the right place and at the right time. My high school teachers were there at such a time as that. They challenged, pushed, and even encouraged me to do a little more than what I considered to be my best. They were great!

I have always kept my focus on what I think is important. Life is too fleeting to be wasted on trivialities and nonsense. From the word go, I told myself I would keep uppermost in my mind the things relevant to nursing. What subjects should I spend more time mastering even in high school? The sciences, English, and mathematics were among the most important, so I concentrated most of my time and effort in mastering those subjects. I forced myself to study Spanish and geography because I didn't have much choice, not realizing that those subjects would become useful and relevant in the future. It never dawned on me that I would one day thank my high school geography teacher for introducing me to North America. I rebelled openly when I had to study about the famous chinook winds, the Trans-Canada Highway, the Rocky Mountains, the prairies, and so many other *irrelevant* things at that stage of my life. I later had the grand pleasure of actually living on the prairies and traveling on the never-ending bridges and train lines on the Trans-Canada Highway! I never also realized how popular and important Spanish would become in my nursing profession even though I have not retained enough Spanish to save my life if the need ever arose!

Time is such an impostor! It sometimes gives false consolation to those who think they are young and have a lot of it in their favor, it goes by so quickly for those who have a mission to accomplish, and it drags on for the bored and indecisive. My time in high school seemed to be on eagle's wings. It raced along every day toward the finish line—the line that would take me closer to realizing my dream.

But four years in burgundy and white uniforms were long enough for me. God is good all the time, so He allowed me to pass the subjects needed in the General Certificate of Education (GCE) examination to be accepted into a school of nursing. (GCE is a British examination given to high school students in ordinary and advanced levels. It is set by both London and Cambridge Universities in Great Britain.) Graduation weekend finally came. It was time to take my leave and say goodbye to my teachers whose positive influence and example had prepared me for the wider world of education. I was humbly proud to have been nominated "Student of the Year." The title came with an all-expense paid one-week trip to the beautiful island of Grand Cayman.

I convinced myself that after four years of hard mental and physical labor I had earned the right to have a little free time to regroup and relax, and so I did just that. A few weeks after graduation, some friends and I took a trip to the famous botanical gardens in Kingston known as The Hope Gardens. In those days, to me, it was a miniature Garden of Eden. Caged reptiles, animals, birds, local and imported, plants and flowers all coexisted to create simple beauty and pleasure for those who chose to appreciate it.

Talk about a God who does things in His own time and in His own way! While there in the garden, I saw folks whom I had not seen for many years. Among those were two of my sister's friends. They were in their final year of nursing school, and they had their textbooks open studying amid the backdrop of paradise. As I stated earlier, I have this nosy streak in me, so I asked them a few questions. God sent those two young ladies to provide me with the roadmap, vehicle, and catalyst I needed to make my entry into the nursing profession. They furnished me with the name and address of the school of nursing in which they were enrolled. I could not wait to return home to start the application process. I never thought for one moment that that simple encounter with those two young ladies was just coincidental. I really believe that this came about because of divine intervention and God's perfect timing!

I prayed to God to give me the correct words to write on the blank piece of paper lying before me. I didn't want to sound too desperate or overzealous, but at the same time I really needed to make a good impression on whoever would chance to read the simple expressions of my heart. I discarded a few sheets of paper before I was happy with the finished essay. Then I neatly folded the paper and placed it into an envelope. This was very serious business! Off to the post office I walked some two miles away because I wanted to be sure, very sure, that I saw that precious piece of mail being placed in the mailbox by no one else but me.

The waiting game began. A famous singer recorded this song some time ago that I love very much, "Every moment's a day, Every day seems a lifetime ... Let me show you the way to a joy beyond compare."

That was exactly what the following days seemed like, a lifetime. Would the director of nursing reply or would she just toss that sheet of paper into the dustbin? Later I chided myself for harboring such negative thoughts. Hadn't I prayed to God from my earliest years that if it be His will then He should open every door and clear every obstacle that might block my way of attaining my dream?

One of the most important letters to grace that post office finally arrived one day! At long last, I got a taste of the desire of my heart. I was given a date and time to sit for a pre-entrance test for acceptance into the school of nursing. I began to envision myself *there*, and I knew where *there* was. My father's vision was rubbing off on me and causing all sorts of pleasure inducing hormones to flow freely through my bloodstream.

Chapter Four

Pre-entrance Test

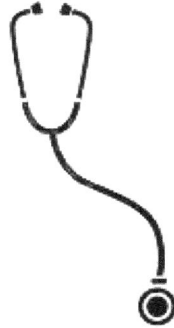

Monday dawned clear and bright, one of those days when it felt great to be alive. I woke up with a song in my heart because I knew something good was about to happen. I prayed to God to keep me calm and sane. I was standing at the very border of the "Promised Land," and I didn't want to block the entrance. I told God I needed an extra dose of wisdom, not as much as He gave to King Solomon, but very close to his. If He gave me even one percent then I stood a good chance of passing because Solomon was the wisest man who ever lived. Toward the end of Solomon's life he became a cynical, depressed, old man, but that is another story! It seems like his favorite quotation was, "Vanity of vanities, all is vanity!" He also wrote this immortal statement, "Let us hear the conclusion of the whole matter, fear God and keep His commandments, for this is the whole duty of man."

My father, God rest his soul, accompanied me to the examination center. All along the way he tried to keep me optimistic and upbeat. He always applied and utilized the power of positive thinking so on that Monday morning I got an extra dose. Imagine using the term dose so matter-of-factly, not realizing that that word would become a part of my vocabulary for the next several years. Isn't life one continuous maze of twists and turns, intrigue, cliffhangers, and adventure? One never knows what lies next around the bend, but it is gratifying to be assured that there is Someone who knows just what is good for us, and that Someone does things independently. I owe all my successes, past and present, to God.

The forty-five mile ride from home to the center ended. I was ushered into a hall that seemed like a place for trying criminal cases and weighing hard facts. There were fifty or so other hopefuls as myself in the room. I guess each of us had our own private agenda. I heard deafening sighs, hissing of teeth, and nervous little coughs as the director of nursing made her appearance at last. She seemed like a foe not to be reckoned with. A military stance was what she wore, and she wore it well.

Introduction of the invigilator, brief instructions, and distributing the papers signaled that the die was cast, and we were either going to sink or swim. I, at that time, told myself I was going to float if that was the last thing I ever did! We were given an Intelligent Quotient (IQ), mathematics, English, and comprehension tests. We also had to complete an essay on "Why I want to be a nurse." Memories of first grade came back like a flood. I assured myself that if I hadn't blown it at that time I stood a pretty good chance of putting some good reasons on paper the second time around.

In a relatively short period of time, I had completed everything but the essay. In all my years of taking examinations and tests, I was always instructed by the invigilators when to begin the next subject. It sounded something like this: "Time is up for mathematic, you may begin the comprehension portion." As a creature of habit, I decided to wait for instructions. I found it quite strange that so long a time period would have elapsed before that instruction was given. I still had lots of time left on my hands, or so I thought!

I mentioned earlier of how time can be an impostor. To this day, I cannot explain why I believed that such an instruction was forthcoming! Maybe I should have pleaded temporary insanity. Time came to an end, and I did not have an essay to turn in. My hopes were dashed, and I scolded myself for being such an idiot. My lifetime dream was then like the proverbial castle in the air or like a fool's paradise. But I was not about to sit and see the castle come crumbling down on my life. I was going to grab the bull by the horns and fight with every ounce of courage I could muster. I did some quick thinking, and I confronted the director. My intent was to plead for leniency and concession.

I introduced myself to her, expecting that she would at least, even for the courtesy of it, acknowledge my presence, but instead, she just kept on walking. I was right at her heels. In my attempt to justify my action, I was given the assurance that if the other forty-nine candidates didn't write the essay then I stood a pretty good chance of hearing from her soon. I told her that that chance seemed very remote. Then I gathered mental ammunition to do battle with her. I remembered something my father used to say: "Never contend with anyone who has nothing to lose!" And she had nothing to lose. So I relaxed and allowed God to fight the battle for me. I had no other recourse.

Then I said to her, "I am quite sure the other young ladies who sat for the test with me did not make that omission. You see Miss Director, all my life it has been my only dream to become a nurse. Today I came this close to realizing it. Now you listen to me, if it's God's will that I should become one, then you will be powerless to stand in my way. To err is human. Thanks for giving me the chance to be here. Have a very pleasant day."

She folded her arms, looked at me, and walked away. I was sure, very sure that the message hit home. A calm enveloped me at that time which was hard to describe. I slept like a baby that night, but I wondered if she did.

It came as no surprise to me, however, that in less than two weeks I received a letter from the nursing school. I wondered what this communication was all about. There was just one way of finding out; I had to open it!

"Dear Ms. McCalla, you are scheduled for an interview on ... at ...." It has been many years since that time. The time and date have long been forgotten, but the euphoria lives on. I knew for sure that God had a hand in all that transpired. It is said that the pen is mightier than the sword. Had I used that pen that day who knows for sure if I would have chopped down every chance of using a syringe or giving a dose of medication to a real, breathing human being! The misunderstanding was a real blessing in disguise.

Chapter Five

The Interview

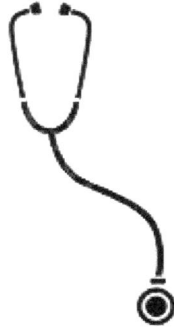

I was given a second chance to prove my mettle. Common sense dictated that because of the fact that I hadn't written the real reason why I would be deemed worthy of becoming a part of this noble profession somewhere in the interview the question would somehow come up. I did a bit of a rehearsal in my mind, pretending that I was just talking to one person, the director. But to my surprise, two persons showed up along with her. I felt as though I was being placed in a den of starving lions! Two matrons from neighboring hospitals were there to decide my fate. Matrons are hospital bigwigs in that part of the world.

"So, Miss McCalla, we are meeting again eh!" remarked the director of nursing.

"I knew that we would," I replied. She smiled, introduced the members of the firing squad, and began the interview. Their demure put me quite at ease.

Just as I had envisioned, the question was asked.

"Tell us, Miss McCalla, in your own words why you want to become a nurse."

My well-rehearsed speech soon took wings and left me speechless and tongue-tied, but not for long. God must have sent a second set of angels to give me clarity of mind and free speech. My tongue and mind knew that this was an emergency situation, so they cooperated very well. Thoughts began to flow like a stream in a desert.

"I want the very best for myself as a person, and I am sure that the nursing profession will be a means of getting me there. Nursing is a noble profession, and when I am trained, I know I will be able to, as much as is humanly possible, to educate people regarding the laws of health and how to prevent disease. I will also help to alleviate pain and, best of all, just be there for them as my patients."

There was silence for a while. That raised a red flag as far as I was concerned. Did I run off too much with my mouth? The spoken word cannot be retrieved no matter how hard one tries. The eraser and delete buttons were invented to correct errors. I had none of those gadgets, only faith that God would translate my speech into eloquence that it would sound like music to the ears of the powers that be!

To my astonishment, the director of nursing said to the other ladies present, "This is the young lady I spoke to you about." I then wondered what on earth she had said about me—that I was the one who committed the sin of omission and told her off quite nicely that fateful morning some weeks before.

"Miss McCalla, your case is unique, and so is your answer. Most times all I hear from candidates applying for nursing is how much they want to help suffering humanity when all they end up doing is to help humanity suffer! You were quite honest in saying that you want a better life for yourself. We all do, and there is nothing wrong with that. Take care of yourself first, then you will be better able to take care of the needs of others, including sick folks."

I felt good, very good!

Then they asked me to stand up so they could look at me—I felt as if I was on the auction block. But those were the days of miniskirts, and they were looking for professional nurses, not models with "BBC," as I called miniskirts, that is, bottoms barely covered. The wearers would make the beholders' minds run amok! I made sure to wear a modest length skirt. I almost did the catwalk like professional models showing off my appropriate skirt. They nodded with approval that the length was just right.

My curiosity was still further aroused as I pondered the reason why I was given a second chance. The answer was supplied soon enough.

"Miss McCalla, you scored very high on the IQ, mathematics, English, and comprehension tests, so I thought that if you told us orally the reasons why you wanted to become a nurse, then you could redeem yourself."

"Redeemed how I love to proclaim it" is one of my favorite hymns, and I thought about that song when she said those words. I knew I was on my way to a brighter tomorrow.

"By the way, Miss McCalla, how do you spell your first name?" asked the director of nursing.

"Millicent," I replied.

"Are you aware that right here on your birth certificate, your name is spelled with only one 'l'—Milicent. Do you also realize that your name is quite unique? For legal purposes, you have to make a conscious effort to use what is written right here. Young lady, you will be hearing from us soon, good luck."

Their smiles spoke loudly. My dream was taking shape right before my very eyes, and I felt exceedingly pleased.

Chapter Six

Complete Physical and Beyond

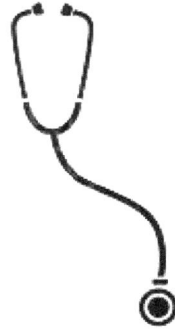

The director of nursing kept her promise of keeping in touch with me. That promise could have gone either way, negatively or favorably. I praised God that I was accepted to start my training in one of the oldest nursing institutions in my country. *So far so good*, I told myself.

But then the physical examination came. I never quite expected to submit a specimen to a laboratory that I believed only the owner should handle with discretion and in the privacy of his or her own bathroom, but it was a requirement. I got a wake-up call because little did I realize that for the rest of my professional life, I would be asking patients to do the same. You see, "What goes around, comes around," as the popular saying goes.

Questions, personal and private, were hurled at me, but I was woman enough to answer them as best as possible. On top of that I was instructed by the doctor to relax and just breathe every few minutes. I am sure my heart and lungs were revved up!

I survived the ordeal quite well and was later instructed to pick up my uniform material across the street. Blue and white would be my attire five days a week for three long years, except for brief vacation periods. Everything was falling into place like a jigsaw puzzle with a picturesque view. I boarded the bus and headed home with free uniform material, the prospect of free housing, and a stipend for the greater part of my training, which was a godsend. All I needed to do was just show up, study hard, and follow the rules.

The rules were a little shy of what was expected from persons serving in the country's armed services. I later confessed that it felt as if I had been to boot camp for three long years. I was taught, however, that discipline and hard work paid rich dividends.

When I reached my destination that afternoon, I alighted from the bus and attempted to cross to the other side of the street while the bus was still parked. I looked in one direction only. But a motor vehicle traveling in the opposite direction was right in my path. Had I gone a few more centimeters into the street, or if the oncoming vehicle had had another thin coat of paint on it, I would have been seriously injured or killed instantly! It seemed as if I was pulled back by unseen hands. There were just a few centimeters between me and instant death. I felt a cool wind across my nose. It must have been the quivering of angels' wings!

Then reality set in. I had a rude awakening, actually. In all of my preparation to face the challenges of the future as a registered nurse, nothing quite prepared me to face death. My focus, or fantasy, was to save lives, and I almost lost mine. I realized then, as I had never done before, the frailty and unpredictability of life. I was young, full of zeal and good intentions, but I was inexperienced in so many things.

As I walked away from that near-death experience, I asked God to be my guide and to help me to remain calm and dependent on Him at all times. Then I thought about the song my father sang when he was down or stressed—"Calm me my God and keep me calm." My family would meet each morning to sing and pray together before dispersing for the day. It was a mini choir, each contributing to a rich, wholesome, homemade melody. Papa would sing bass, my mother soprano, and the rest of us would just sort of find a slot in between. So I adapted my father's prescription for calm and serenity, and decided to sing that song.

Even today in my profession I use that song in every emergency, and it works all the time. I was about to wade into deep, uncharted waters, and I needed all the right maps and compass that would bring me to a safe haven. The only Guide I knew then as well as now is God.

The long awaited day finally came for me to leave the comfort zone of my home and check into a hostel that would be another home away from home for me for two years. My uniforms were made and nicely pressed. I was given a list of must-haves. One of the dare-not-do-without items was a pair of surgical scissors. Drilled into my head from day one until September 11, 2001, was, "A good nurse always travels with her pair of scissors." That very first pair with which I started nursing school went with me every where until restrictions were placed on airline travelers about carrying anything that might be deemed dangerous, including a pair of scissors. I had to leave that pair behind in Calgary, Canada.

Chapter Seven

Well, This Is It!

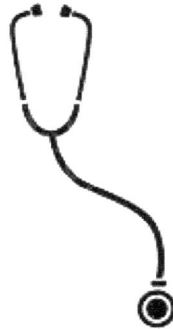

My country's government had purchased a hotel that was later converted into classrooms and a dormitory for student nurses. I was in the company of strangers, but I had often heard that "strangers are friends we have not met," so I decided to meet people and make a few friends. I did not need too many. My roommate happened to be one of the finest human beings imaginable. She was dignified, brilliant, and considerate. We respected each other's boundaries and privacy and were supportive of each from the very beginning of our training.

For the longest time, maybe even since the inception of the nursing institution, the training was based on the "apprenticeship" program. Student nurses were given a lot of responsibilities and expected to keep up with long clinical hours, and at the same time, they had to study very hard. To me, it was a type of cheap labor masked in professionalism. Many of these overworked graduates were pretty well burnt out by the time the program was done. After many years of following this type of training program, some wise individuals decided to infuse new life into the old system. The solution was called "The Two Plus One Programme."

This new system entailed that we were given complete student status. For the first two years we would be in a structured classroom environment combining theory and practical skills in nursing. We were first given hands-on training by the faculty in the classroom; then later we applied those skills in the respective clinical areas we were assigned to. I found this new approach very practical and tailored to our needs as student nurses.

We were evaluated every step of the way. Let's face it, we could not afford to fail because the very future of this new system rested squarely on our shoulders. We were like guinea pigs dressed in blue and white, but I loved it! After a period of two years, we were ready to sit for the qualifying examination set by my country's Council of Nursing, the equivalent of the state boards in North America. We later had to do a one-year internship in all the areas covered by the curriculum. We were then given the title of nurse interns.

In my quiet moments I take a backward glance on the long road over which I have traveled, and I cannot help but laugh out loud. On the eve of the start to our training, more than 90 young ladies and senior students assembled in the cafeteria. We were taught how to put our caps together. In those bygone days, nurses were required to wear caps. Our cap was just a piece of fabric that had to be starched to the texture of a board, making it very rigid! The undersurface was moistened, threaded through, and then pulled together to form the cap. I think we called this work of art "fluting," Why am I telling you all this? Well, all I know is this, if that cap was not ready and *"fluted"* come Monday morning, there would be weeping and gnashing of teeth!

Sleep that first Sunday night at the hostel was punctuated with frequent trips to the bathroom as feelings of impending doom as well as great expectation swept over me. I had a barrage of mixed emotions. Why should I be anxious, fearful, and flustered when I had been wishing and hoping and praying for so many years? My dream was just a sunrise away, and there I was panicking! My father's song, "Calm me my God and keep me calm," came to me like a warm security blanket, and I managed to catch a few hours of blissful sleep before morning.

My first day as a student nurse finally dawned. I thought to myself, "Well, this is it." There I was on the very fringes of professionalism as well as fear of the unknown. Not everyone always embraces change, and it was quite obvious that the new program was not welcomed by some doctors as well as nurses. Resentment was felt all around, but as a group, we were resolute to beat the odds and succeed at all cost.

Close to one hundred students started the course, and it was predicted that by its completion not half of that number would remain. We assembled in the auditorium and were greeted by the school's faculty and the parliamentary secretary from the Ministry of Health. After brief formalities and small talk, the parliamentarian strutted to the podium. I remember her speech as though it was uttered just a few minutes ago. She titled it "Strive for Excellence." A hush fell over the crowded auditorium. How well I remember bits and pieces of her speech, enough to actually cite her.

"Ladies and gentlemen, nursing is an art and a science. You must daily strive for excellence."

She then gave an analogy of a secretary typing and making errors. The secretary would delete or erase as the case might be or just toss that piece of paper into the dustbin. Then she drove the point home.

"If a nurse gives a patient the wrong medication, performs the wrong procedure on him or her, chances are that error could cause permanent damage or even prove fatal. You have to strive for excellence every day of your professional life. Nursing demands the highest standard of performance. You cannot afford to make mistakes!" She rattled on for many minutes.

Without any apology, she told us that by the end of the course just a handful of us would graduate. She also tried to console us that it was not too late to reconsider our decision to start the training. This woman actually offered cash for transportation to anyone who wished to leave. My roommate of a few hours gave me a look of hopelessness. Her eyes spoke louder than her words. She needed just a push to accept the money and run far away from that place. Our eyes were engaged in combat, and I was determined to win at all cost. I spoke to her as if I were a professional ventriloquist—"You are going nowhere. You and I are going to finish this course if it's the last thing I do!"

A smile came over her face like the rays of the sun breaking through after a stormy night.

I told myself that if one student was to complete the course then that student would be me, and I planned to do just about anything, ethically, to prove the parliamentarian wrong. I believed she was just using a very bad case of reverse psychology to scare the living daylights out of us! I told myself also that there would be a major blizzard in my tropical paradise before I would allow her to detour me from my dream by even one iota!

Have you ever gone to a church service where the preacher delivered a "hell-and-brimstone" sermon in which you saw yourself as the vilest sinner bound for the bottomless reaches of eternal hell? Then he calls for all the sinners to march up to the front and confess their evil doings and repent before they even think of leaving that church. That was exactly how I felt after she finished her revival-type lecture. There were many a tearful eye in that place that hot Monday morning. For a brief moment I was totally disorientated to time, place, and person. I didn't know if I was in a church or a school or who was talking. Was it a preacher, an evangelist, or a parliamentarian?

Later that morning we were given a royal tour of the hospital where we would spend the greater part of our training. I really believe that everything that transpired in those few hours was a deliberate attempt to make or break us. I saw for the first time in my life dressings on ulcers that badly needed to be changed. Dirty bedpans and pain and despair all passed in slow motion before my very eyes. The reality of it all began to sink into place.

"So this is nursing!" I told myself.

Lunchtime came at last. For lunch, we had a choice of fish or fish or fish! We could either take it or leave it. My stomach told me to take it, but my mind said, "Oh no!" The color and look of the fish brought back vivid memories of the ulcers I had just seen a couple of minutes before. I dashed to the bathroom and negotiated with my stomach not to empty its contents. It compromised a bit. Strange as it might seem, I was not the only person having that problem. Quite a few girls headed to the bathroom as well. That fish, I am quite sure, did the trick! I told myself that the situation I was then facing could not get any worse, so it had to get better and fast if I was to maintain my sanity and not lose sight of my dream.

Chapter Eight

First Day of Training

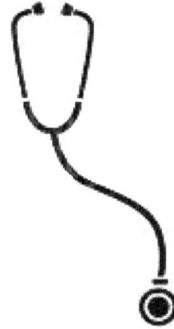

On the very first day in a structured classroom setting, we were given an introduction to nursing.

The International Council of Nursing defines nursing as "encompass[ing] autonomous and collaborative care of individuals of all ages, families, groups and communities sick or well in all settings. Nursing includes the promotion of health, prevention of illness, and the care of ill disabled and dying people. Advocacy, promotion of safe environment, research, participation in shaping health policy and in patient and health systems management and education are also key nursing roles."

We were also taught that it is an art and science. The basic principles, concepts, and practices of nursing were taught from the very beginning. Anybody can hand out a bedpan, give a sponge bath, or even make a bed, but a nurse is taught the rationale and the method, and all this is done with the comfort of the patient in mind. This principle makes a big difference. Everything I learned from that day forward was hinged on knowledge, skill, and commonsense. That was to me the fundamental of nursing.

The first practical skill I learned was how to make an unoccupied bed. I had been making my own bed from childhood, so I wondered why I should be *taught* to make a bed. Just grab hold of a sheet, give it a good shake and throw the thing over the bed then tuck the loose ends firmly under the mattress. What's the big deal? Was I in for a surprise! Shake sheets, tuck loose ends under the mattress, and forget about it? Not so! Hang on to your seats, or sheets. This routine chore was a skill that had to be mastered under the watchful eyes of the sister tutors, otherwise known as instructors, professors, or nurse educators.

White seems to be the color of choice for sheets in most, if not all, hospitals. Why? I have never gotten the real reason, but I am still researching it. So there we were with the tools with which to work: sheets, draw sheet, waterproof mattress cover, pillows, and pillowcases. So far, so good; this should be easy!

"Body mechanics" was a new word that was to become a part of our vocabulary for the rest of our profession life. We had to apply "good body mechanics" from the word go. We were taught how to lift patients and heavy objects using our center of gravity by maintaining a wide base with our legs while keeping our backs straight, thus minimizing strain and pressure on our backs and necks. "No bending from the waist, bend your knees instead, get close to the object you are lifting and maintain good posture." That was a law that had to be obeyed! After many years of using the big muscles of my arms and legs, those poor body parts are crying out for mercy as well as revenge! "Enough is enough" they seem to be saying!

Body mechanics was demonstrated.

"Now you try!" was the command by the sister tutor. We were self-conscious students, but we tried to convince the tutor that her few minutes of instruction had not been in vain; we had some amount of nursing material hidden someplace under those blue and white uniforms! We all would eventually master the art.

After that exercise we were told, "Now let me show you how to make an unoccupied bed while *maintaining good body mechanics*." I thought to myself that I would literally scream if I heard that term one more time.

"Now remember this, do not shake the sheet unnecessarily. Gently unfold it a little at a time. Cover half of the bed, then put on your waterproof cover and draw sheet. Go to the head of the bed and tuck the sheet under the mattress. Now go to the foot of the bed, grab the loose end of the sheet, and tuck it in to secure your corners. Stretch the rest of the sheet until it is wrinkle-free. Go to the other side of the bed and repeat what you just did. Take hold of your pillow, bend it in half, and gently insert it into the pillowcase. Turn the opened end of the pillow away from the door."

The end product of that bed making was like fine art.

"What a hassle!" I grunted to myself. It was like folding and unfolding a country's national flag.

After mastering the art of making an unoccupied bed, the next level was to make one with a live human being in it. Basically the same principle applied, except that we had to be conscious of the fact that a human being was there who needed all the privacy and dignity that he or she deserved. As the days and weeks progressed, we began to do more "fun things" such as giving and receiving bedpans the proper way; collecting stool, urine, and sputum specimen; emptying emesis basins; doing bed baths; cleaning dentures; feeding patients; and getting them in and out of bed using "good body mechanics!"

One time I saw one of my classmates who had just retrieved a full bedpan from a patient handling it as if she were a waitress with a tray heading to a table to serve champagne and caviar. I just prayed that whatever was in that bedpan would be merciful to her! Donning a pair of gloves or using a mask were not very popular or essential in doing those "fun things" in those days. A couple minutes of good hand washing was mostly what we did.

Later we practiced changing wound dressings using sterile techniques. Our tutors were uncompromising with us in that regard. Then we picked up speed in researching drugs, better known as medications. Pharmacology was one of the most challenging areas of nursing for me, and it still is. When I read about the side effects of so many drugs that we give to our patients, I think to myself, those meds are like weapons of mass destruction! But nevertheless, the benefits of most of those medications most times far outweigh their risks. But until we get to the stage where we eat right, obey the laws of nature, control our weight, and live healthy productive lives, then we will just have to swallow our cupful of medications to stay alive.

The essence of nursing is doing for the patient that which he cannot do for himself independently. We got that drilled into our heads from the very start of our training. As the days faded into weeks, we took turns practicing on one another, thus reinforcing what we were taught until we became more proficient. I still remember the thrill I experienced the first time I was addressed as "nurse!" I innocently asked, "Who me?"

"Yes, you, young lady. You are now a student nurse so never forget it." At that point I felt like a big shot. Nurse indeed, eh! After a while I began to respond to my newfound title spontaneously.

Chapter Nine

My First Injection and First Expiration

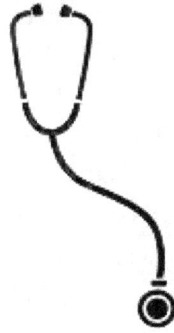

Over the years people have changed the name of injections to shots, inoculations, boosters, while others try to make it sound like no big deal—it's just a little mosquito sting—but it is still a patient's greatest nightmare. No matter how you say it, an injection is the introduction of a sharp, hollow, slender piece of metal into a person's body in order to administer medication through an attached syringe. Administering it has become second nature to me over the years, but I cannot and will never forget the first time I gave an injection to a living, breathing human being. That was a planned trauma!

We were taught the sites and the rationale for using those areas of the body for administering injections. In those days, antibiotics were not in such abundance. We maintained sterility and clean techniques in most every area of practice. That, I believe, minimized the need for a lot of antibiotics both in duration and frequency. Well, the first injection I gave was penicillin. It came in a phial and in powdered form. A day or two before that fateful day, we were given hands-on training using an orange. I was a pro in attaching the needle to the syringe, pulling up the fluid from a phial, and giving the poor orange "juice"! I mercilessly poked that fruit. If the dear orange had had a voice, it would have used a few choice words. I knew what I was doing. I was confident, oh so very confident! In fact, I could teach the sister tutor a thing or two when it came to giving injections!

The rule of thumb when administering any form of treatment or medication is to know the right person, the right time, the right medication and dosage, and the right route. If any of those things are overlooked, chances are that great damage might result. We as nurses and other healthcare professionals cannot afford to make any form of error. You can't amputate the wrong limb or take out the wrong organ, and then say, "Oops, I made a boo-boo. I am so sorry. I am only human. Mistakes do happen you know. I hope you understand. Let bygones be bygones." That does not sit right in any clinic, hospital, or private practice or with any patient or their families. Now back to the first needle.

I got the patient's chart, or docket as it was called in those days, checked the doctor's order, and prepared the right drug, right dose, route, and time. I had all the required stuff. Dread gripped my very soul! This was the first time I, the "pro," mixed *real* penicillin with *real* sterile water in a *real* phial, drew it up in a *real* sterile syringe, got rid of *real* air in the syringe, approached a *real* patient, and asked him if he knew who he *really* was! I wanted to run away from that man's bedside as far as the east is from the west.

"Now, nurse, tell me how you calculate the dosage of the medication, the amount of sterile water you need to dissolve the powder in the phial, and show me what you are going to do next," said the sister tutor.

I always brag about my God because, you see, I cannot remember a time when I ever needed Him and He was not there for me. He is my Jehovah-jireh, the God who always sees, who always provides! I don't call these moments coincidental; I call them divine interventions. The good Lord knew that at that moment, I needed a timeout, so He distracted my tutor by having someone call her on the telephone, and He made sure that she had a long conversation with that individual at the other end of the line.

You might remember the student nurses I met at the botanical gardens that Sunday who gave me the name and address of the nursing school. Well, one of them, then a senior, happened to be passing by when she saw me and came over to greet me. She hadn't the foggiest idea I was actually in training. It was a wonderful encounter, and I got a chance to thank her for the part she had played in my life thus far. She immediately sensed my predicament and solved the problem for me stat. With a sense of urgency, she immediately solved my problem! That young lady was an angel sent in human form, stat!

The conversation on the phone lasted the right length of time. I was one step ahead of this sister tutor. Courage, that was what I needed to convince myself that I could indeed implement the information I had learned.

"Okay, nurse McCalla, let me see you instill the sterile water into the phial and then aspirate," my boss said. That was the litmus test for me. I began to use all the mental power I possessed but never knew existed to concentrate and tell myself that the big shot standing there breathing fire down my neck was only a woman like myself!

So let the show begin! I thought. *Syringe, needle, sterile water, phial, here I come. If you are not ready, then I will just have to start without you! Come on hands; stop shaking for heaven's sake. Adrenal glands, slow down a bit so that my heartbeat can get the hint. Sweat glands take a hike because if you don't, then this uniform is going to need some very hot tropical sunshine to dry it real fast. Dear God, what did I get myself into?*

In that midsummer tropical heat wave, my body parts and functions totally ignored my pep talk. I was then ready to use the fight or flight mechanism, which I later learned really exist. Sweat began running down my back and face like Niagara Falls.

In spite of my body not cooperating, my mind remained in charge, and I managed to draw up the penicillin into the syringe. Now for the final hurdle!

"Nurse, let's go to the patient and administer the medication," commanded my boss. Today, for patient safety, healthcare professionals are required to ask patients to state their name and date of birth and make sure that the information matches the ID band affixed to the patients' wrist. In those days, it was not mandatory, but nonetheless, it was important. I went up to the very quiet, innocent looking gent, introduced myself, and told him of my mission, which sounded something like this:

"Mr. Brown, my name is Milicent McCalla, and I am a student nurse. This is my sister tutor, and she is going to be with me while I give you your injection." My own voice sounded strange and faraway.

"Nurse, are you ready?" If the truth be known, she sounded just as nervous as I. After all, if I goofed up, her reputation and license were pretty much on the line. I did not have any of those commodities to lose at that point in time.

"Yes, I am ready," I replied.

"What are you waiting for?" she asked. I had apparently paused too long for her liking.

"Nothing," I answered.

After what seemed like an eternity, I mustered the courage to push away stupidity and timidity and look to God for help. My dad's song, "Calm me my God and keep me calm," came to me at a time when I needed it most.

Milicent, take a deep breath, relax, and be assured that God is with you, and you will be okay. That was the reassurance I received as I changed my focus and attitude.

"Mr. Brown, kindly pull down your pajamas. Thank you. I am going to clean your skin with alcohol. It is going to feel a little cool. Okay, Mr. Brown, try to relax while I put this needle right here in your hip."

I will never forget that man's eyes. It was a look of pity for me and for himself, and they haunted me for a long time. I didn't cause any obvious injury to the poor gentleman. He was able to walk and talk after I was finished with him. He even thanked me and wished me good luck in my training. What a sweetheart! After that first attempt, I could hardly wait for more opportunities to give injections! As a matter of fact, I always made myself available to test new procedures.

One day a patient was brought into the ward. He was unresponsive and extremely dirty and grimy. It appeared that the streets had been his residence for a very long time. Anyway, when he arrived on the ward, three of us student nurses volunteered to transform this man into Mr. Clean. That was a mammoth task, indeed. He had layers and layers of dirt caked to his skin and hair, but that did not deter us one bit. After many basins of warn soapy water, the mud began to fade away, exposing skin I am sure he had not seen in many years. We applied lotion and powdered his skin, and he looked like a brand new English penny straight from the Royal Mint!

We stood back and admired what we had just done, feeling quite good about ourselves. With our mission now accomplished, we placed him between clean white sheets and gave him a pair of brand new pajamas. The three of us couldn't stop bragging about how we had transformed this man into the epitome of loveliness. We took turns fussing over him. But strange as it might sound, in less than an hour after his transformation, the patient expired, dead as a doornail! Maybe we washed him too clean. The pores might have been opened up too rapidly and the poor man's heart and lungs could not handle it. This is sheer speculation, of course!

The most important thing to us at that point was that he died with some measure of dignity. Later we wrapped his body in a clean white sheet and sent him to the morgue in fine style. No tears were shed, but we wondered if he had any loved ones to miss him. That was just the foretaste of what nursing is all about. We try to save lives, but we never know when we will have to deal with death.

Chapter Ten

Fearfully and Wonderfully Made

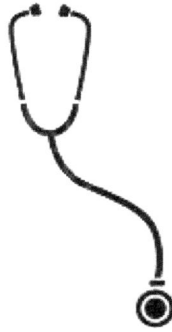

In the short time I had been in training, I believed I was mastering the fundamentals of nursing quite well. I then entered a new and exciting phase of my education in which I saw things I never thought existed. One of the things that delighted me most was the structure and function of the human body. Every day I became more enlightened regarding the awesome, intelligently designed human body and how each part is interdependent on the other. Back in high school, I had learned basic biology, but this was so detailed!

Anatomy and physiology revealed to me the awesomeness of a God who did not randomly make us but made us special and one of a kind. We might look like someone else, but each of us is so unique, it's just amazing and wonderful. We skimmed the surface of genetic coding, the means by which DNA and RNA molecules carry genetic information in living cells. That information is still Greek to me! It made no sense to me then, but I could appreciate the fact that we are fearfully and wonderfully made by an awesome and loving God.

I also determined that the human body is like a very close-knit family. When one member becomes ill, the whole family is affected, and some members of the family try to compensate by working overtime, sometimes even at the others' expense, until that member improves or recovers. I also learned that there is a closeness of the mind and body and that a positive upbeat attitude make all the difference in the life of an individual. I also learned that hope and a reason to live in spite of the odds sustain people in difficult times.

I was also deeply amazed at the body's ability to heal and repair itself. I became familiar with how bones mend themselves after a fracture and the process by which blood clots after we get a cut so that we do not bleed to death. I learned about the body's great filtration system. I observed patients who suffered from some type of neurological conditions respond favorably to medication and physiotherapy. Just the reaction of the patient's pupil to light, movement of a finger or a limb, or the ability to squeeze someone's hands or swallow encouraged everyone involved in the case that life was still in the body and that better days were ahead. I learned about the body's ability to regenerate certain organs and tissues. If a lobe of a good liver is removed for whatever reason that structure has the ability to regenerate itself over time.

I got a pleasant surprise the first time I visited the operating room. The human body is exquisitely beautiful on the inside in spite of our outward flaws. The colors displayed on the inside are hard to capture on canvas. I found beauty in unexpected places, and I felt humble and grateful to be made a human being. God could have made me a dog or a cow or a bird, but He chose to make me in His image, smart and intelligent and with a mind to choose. I observed that the organs, glands, and intestines were neatly assembled. No one part is fighting for dominance, status, or position. Each is there doing what it was designed to do. So many shades of color yet no discrimination. Internally each nerve, tissue, cell, and the other structures that come together to make us individuals, coexist peacefully in their limited space. What wonderful lessons we can learn and apply to our outward environment!

Among God's fondest wishes for us is that we be in good health and be happy. We all have a significant part to play in maintaining optimum health and preventing illnesses and diseases. Sometimes, try as hard as we possibly can, unexplained diseases still overtake us, but we just have to keep doing the right thing and hope for the best.

I often laugh at the dozens of diseases my classmates and I had during our training—you name it, we had it! It all goes to show how closely linked our minds and bodies are. Even stranger was the speed at which we recovered from these illnesses. Each time we studied a disease, someone was sure to experience some symptoms of that particular disease. At first I never mentioned the "diseases" I was having lest I be a case study by the student body. To my surprise, someone made mention of the fact that she felt she had the disease we had just studied. Upon her admission, a chorus of responses rang out, "Me too, I have the same problem!"

When our stomachs hurt, then surely we had some sort of peptic ulcer. If our right side ached, then we had appendicitis and needed emergency surgery. If we had a headache longer than what we deemed normal and if it was accompanied by dizziness, then the neurologist and brain surgeon needed to be consulted stat because we had some type of space occupying lesion in our brains that was pressing on some vital areas and had to be removed as quickly as possible! We had all types of cancers from breast to colon. If it were possible, some of us girls would have had enlarged prostate glands! Some of us in our late teens and early twenties were menopausal if we felt a bit flushed even in our upper eighty-degree tropical climate. We blamed it on hormone imbalance and needed hormone replacement! As new diseases were introduced, then the original ones just seemed to spontaneously resolve themselves. Why waste precious time nursing those when there were more fancy ones to contract? I remember how quickly my intestinal obstruction was relieved with a glass of prune juice, increased oral fluids, and a quick trip to the bathroom. I convinced myself that it was nothing short of a miracle!

I realized that suddenly, simple everyday words and phrases began taking on new names. For practically all my life, going to the privacy of my bathroom with the intention of doing what I had to do, followed by Lysol spray, took on fancy terms such as defecation! When I passed gas, it was known as flatus! I usually saw folks with very swollen legs and problems breathing, and kids would sometimes giggle and say, "You see that man over there; his heart is sick. You see how his feet swell up?" That swelling was later named edema! Don't ever call bad breath, bad breath! It was then halitosis! Pink eye was for the layperson. Pink eye got a new title for me—conjunctivitis! Vomiting was called emesis. And the list went on and on.

One day, just for fun, I decided to try out some of my newly acquired vocabulary on my dad. He laughed so loudly that tears streamed from his eyes. He then had the nerve to patronizingly say to me, "If I were still a police officer, I would have you arrested, myself, and send you off to prison for life. Those words sure sound like swear words or foul, obscene language to me! Those words are punishable by law!"

Chapter Eleven

"Every Behavior Is Meaningful"

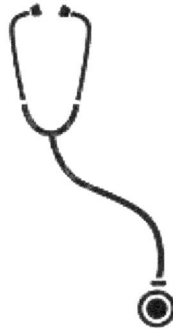

I clearly remember those words, "Every behavior is meaningful." Simply stated, everything an individual does, he or she has a reason for doing it. When I grasped that concept, I began looking at actions. Why am I acting the way I am? What's going on with me? What changes do I have to make to become a better well-rounded individual while I occupy this little spot on planet earth? I was determined to start with me. I still have not found all the answers I am looking for because it seems that the most difficult thing to do is to know one's self completely.

Around this time I was introduced to psychology, and I fell in love with it from the very first class. Later I learned applied sociology and then psychiatry. I was taught that what an individual perceives is happening to him or her at a particular time is more important than what is really happening. In other words, the way I understood this concept is that people's beliefs or perception of things at a certain point in life are quite real to them, although to others it might seem trivial.

Gradually I began to apply those basic concepts to my patients and the people with whom I came in contact. The intent was not to scrutinize or to "shrink" them but to make allowances and adjustments without being judgmental. I also learned to appreciate people's cultures and beliefs and just simply accept them for who they really are. I also learned that there is a very thin line between sanity and insanity and that people's coping skills differ and that people need people.

It seemed as though I had a thirst to learn as much as I could about human behavior. I learned about basic needs that all human beings have and that if those needs are not met, most everything else takes second place. The need for survival, food, water, communication, security, and acceptance and appreciation are more than basic needs, they are *basic rights*! I grasped the concept that the experiences in our formative years in our home environment, coupled with our cultural background and our value system all have a marked impact on what we become later in life.

But in spite of my thirst for knowledge, I had a rude awakening when I first visited a psychiatric hospital. I saw acutely ill psychiatric patients who, over time, were able to return to society as well adjusted citizens. I also saw many who had been there for countless years and seemed to be beyond help. I thought to myself, *Which is worse, a sick mind or a sick body?* If I had to choose one, then give me a sick body any day!

Once a week we had what was called "Unstructured Group Discussion." The whole student body, along with our tutors, would sit in a circle and talk. But the very first time this unexplained event was thrust upon us, we sat there wondering what on earth was going to happen next. I think the whole exercise was to teach us some very interesting things about ourselves. I observed students playing with their hair, crossing and uncrossing their legs, sighing, making faces, doodling, or hissing their teeth in boredom. Some were yawning so much it was unbelievable, and there is no cure for the common yawn! Tension was thick and hostile! Why were we there?

Finally one brave heart could not take the silence any longer, so she spoke. She spoke about a current event taking place that she thought would be of interest to all of us. Gradually others joined in the discussion while the rest of us chose to keep silent. Another person tested the water, so to speak, and others responded, but overall, it was a very awkward situation. For one long hour, we were held hostage by the tutors! No one dared try to leave for any reason! After what seemed like an eternity, the director of nursing spoke.

"Those of you who spoke, why did you do speak, and those who never spoke, why didn't you? Did you want others to hear how well informed you were, how glib you are or what? Were the rest of you just shy or dumb? Look inside yourselves and answer those question. Why were you afraid of silence? Go home and ponder those questions." We all breathed a sigh of relief still dreading what the following weeks would bring.

One great lesson that I learned during that very interesting course, is that we cannot change people, but we can change ourselves one day at a time. Loving and accepting ourselves for all that we really are, makes all the difference to our mental health and wellbeing. Anything else would be a total sham. Life experiences can be crushing or even emotionally traumatic, but I strongly believe that God is able to help us cope. Let nothing stand between us and our dreams. We all need to laugh at adversities, setbacks, misfortune and keep going ahead and grab our dreams by the horn! Some "Impossible dreams" do come true. I am a living proof of this notion!

Chapter Twelve

"Look Out World, Here I Come"

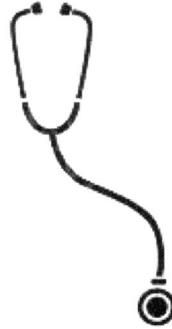

During the part of my training covering midwifery and pediatrics, I came full circle in the knowledge that humans are intelligently designed and not as afterthoughts. We were taught that life begins at conception. Regardless of the way in which that conception occurred, it follows a sequence of events that the mother has very little control over.

Believe it or not, I still have notes I took during midwifery and pediatrics, and those concepts have come in handy even at the point of writing this book. I still have confidence in my sister tutors enough to quote from them more than a quarter of a century later. Granted, some things have changed since the days of the "Pony Express," but the fundamentals of nursing have not changed. Methods of doing things might differ, but the principles remain the same.

A well-planned, welcomed pregnancy begins with Mr. Male Sperm as he flexes his muscles and swims upstream in the race of a lifetime. His very life depends on winning this competition. He outsmarts all the other millions of contestants, and he is the only one worthy of wearing the crown. He is now Lord of the Ring! He unites with a female ovum and the morula stage begins within six days. In rapid succession new names are given like blastocyst stage and trophoblastic stage. This little, bitsy human being has twenty-three pairs of chromosomes and genes from both sides of the family, enough to determine the physical features of the baby.

I found this part of my theoretical training so interesting it was hard to fathom. This is a miracle beyond human comprehension. Within four weeks or so after conception, the eyes, ears, and respiratory system begin to form. By seven weeks fingers like little buds on a tree have formed and soon their own set of fingerprints will emerge. No one can duplicate those fingerprints no matter how one tries. The mold is discarded after it is given! Can you believe it? Eight weeks down the road, its little heartbeat can be heard, and then by nine to twelve weeks, it can move its fingers and even swallow!

Around this time the mom begins to lose her waistline and her hourglass figure. In the future she might not regain it, but the precious little person growing inside of her is worth the loss of the fashion model figure! By the time this precious creation is sixteen to twenty weeks old, it can hear its mother's heartbeat and even music, and it responds to touch. Come six months its sweat glands are functioning, and by seven months it begins to do a bit of aerobics. You should see it stretching and bending and pushing as if it owns the place! It can even hiccup! It is really keeping the mother informed that it is still there, because each time it moves, the mother is very much aware. We call this action quickening.

We have to fast forward the process because there is no way I can go into every detail as to the rapid changes this "big shot" is undergoing in the womb. It is moving so fast I almost forgot to throw in a few new names attached to it like embryo and fetus. By eight months it has put on quite a bit of meat on its bones and its skeleton is fairly hardened. Before that time it had only cartilage, but now it is boasting real bones! This is a period of intense growth. It develops a greasy coating all over its body called vernix caseosa to protect it from excess exposure to the amniotic fluid. It also receives antibodies from its mom to protect it from certain types of infections. This to me is the ultimate type of life support system anyone can receive! The baby puts on an average of half a pound every week until it decides to make its triumphant entry into the world.

As the baby prepares for its grand entrance into the world, it starts to communicate with its mother, as if to say, "Mom, you be very sure to get us to the hospital. Ready or not, here I come!" The mother is smart enough to listen to the command of her baby; she knows that she needs to obey, stat. This word keeps popping up every once in a while because there is urgency and importance attached to it.

This is where I came in with all the drama and big ado! A film was shown a day before highlighting labor and delivery, but what I saw in class never quite prepared me for the actual live performance. A very pregnant woman, two midwives, and I were in the delivery room. Silence reigned. I am an artist, and I think in abstract! I began to see beauty in this unexpected place. I then gave this unborn person a voice and an ear in my imagination.

"Listen up, Mama, I am going to rupture this sack of fluid that has been keeping me protected, yet very restricted. What do you call it? Oh yes, amniotic fluid. Well, I do not need it anymore so give it to somebody else for all I care. Do you see where I now position my head? For the past three weeks or so my head has been suspended downward. This is a very compromising position for me, really. However, if I was sitting as normal people, then we both would be in big trouble! I have been causing you to run to the bathroom more frequently because I am *camping out* close to your bladder. Did you stop to think why this was happening? Your uterus is going to contract painfully. It won't be a piece of cake, but it's all in the game called life."

I flipped back to reality as a contraction formally began. With each contraction the baby's head was pushed further downward. The head internally rotated to pass through what is called the ischial spine. Gradually an opening appeared. Oh yes, the cervix was dilating! Was that a head? It was, indeed, because I saw hair! The contractions became stronger and more frequent. The head emerged at last. With very little assistance from the midwives, I saw what is called external rotation to allow the shoulders to take an "antero-posterio" position, but forget the big words, the boy was coming! The rotation and position allowed the delivery of the full body. I was awestruck and was immediately drawn to this new addition to the earth's population! It was a healthy, baby boy with an Apgar score of ten. This score is used to express the physical condition of a newborn infant. A score of ten is as good as it gets. I didn't wait to have the midwives make that evaluation. I did it myself because that baby seemed perfect at birth. Later the placenta was expelled, and of course the midwives checked to see that it was intact and that no retained products were left inside the mother's body.

I paused in my tracks amid all the excitement and just for a moment pondered what that baby might become in the future. It has been many years since I experienced that miracle, and I often wonder, did I ever see him again as a boy, teenager, young adult, or man? Even if I did, I obviously would have had no idea of who he might have been. I only hope that the world has been kind to him and that he has someone to look up to in a positive way because he got a seemingly good head start physically.

It suddenly dawned on me that only moments before a very pregnant woman, who could not even see her big toes in a standing or lying position, two midwives, and I had been joined in a flash by a fifth person, and my, wasn't he a noisy one too! That young fellow certainly had a good pair of lungs. I wondered what exactly passed through the mind of that young, inexperienced, first-time mom. She wanted that child badly, and she had a seemingly loving husband, so I switched my thoughts to the present time.

That little baby gave out a cry that could not be quelled until he was cleaned up real good and fast and then fed. He was born hungry! He wanted human milk, and he demanded it stat! I guessed that he could be making unuttered statements such as these:

"I am here as I promised. Now, I have some house rules that I intend to lay down! Everything will be fine so long as you obey my commands. Right this minute, put on some of those fancy things you call clothes. You see, where I came from, I had no need of such things. Naked came I into this world, and naked will I return! I am born broke. I am almost like a parasite, totally dependent on a host, and I will remain thus up until age eighteen, or if I push my luck a bit more, I might even hang around until I am twenty-one! I never invited myself here in the first place, so whoever is responsible for my being here had better keep me warm, safe, and secure, and above all, well fed. Human milk is for human babies, and cow's milk is for calves. I demand human milk now straight from the mammary glands, stat! No readymade formula from a bottle for me, no siree. If I suspect that you are neglecting your responsibilities, you will never hear the end of it. I will keep the peace as long as you cooperate with my agenda!"

Thus spoke the new kid on the block! I once bought a bib for one of my nephews with a catchy little wording affixed. "My father is the boss. My mother is his boss, and I am their boss!" Oh, so true!

Over the years I have had the distinct pleasure of seeing young children behaving as children should. There is very little self-consciousness, no one vying for first place, position, or always wanting to be right. There is no harboring of guilt or grudges. Their games are unstructured, and they don't worry about tomorrow. Time is of very little importance to them. They are not as fragile as we adults sometimes make them out to be. They certainly are not made out of crystals or eggshells! When they hug you and plant some wet mushy kisses on your cheek, they hug you straight from the heart with no strings attached. They can be painfully and brutally honest, so as adults, we have to be careful what we do or say in front of these seemingly innocent little angels. If we do not want to have anything echoed, then we can't say it in their hearing!

"Rose, daddy said that he is going to fire you because you can't cook. You burnt up a big chicken yesterday. You can't do anything right!"

"Julie, that's not a nice thing for you to say to her!"

"But auntie, you were standing right there when daddy said those things about her."

I was caught in the crossfire between my innocent little niece and my sister's helper.

One of my nieces, Denise, made a full sentence the first time she decided to try out her tongue, but what she said was quite *fresh* if you please! My brother Noel was put in his place when she said, "You be quiet over there. This is not your house." Everyone was shocked, but she mimicked what she had heard. They echo and mirror everything we do and say. We are an open book from which they learn life's lessons.

Sometimes I get such a kick out of hearing them babble away, unabashed, wide-eyed, and innocent. I get tickled watching them dress up in their parents' clothes. A little girl puts on her mom's three-inch high heel shoes, hat, dress, dark glasses as big as goggles on her little face, and makeup with lips as red as cherries and swears that she is Mae West or Miss America! Then the little chap struggles to put on dad's jacket and tie before diving into dad's size ten pair of shoes. He sneaks into the bathroom, gets dad's shaving cream, empties the whole can on his face and prepares to shave an invisible beard and mustache.

Both girls and boys can be very serious about dressing themselves as they begin to grow more independent. In fact, plenty of children make a big stink if any adult even thinks of lending them a hand. They know exactly what they are doing! Just picture it. They are deep in concentration, tongue sticking out, two legs in one pant leg, right shoe on left foot, left foot in right shoe, shirt on backwards, and buttons missing their holes, but they know what they are doing! What a sight for sore eyes! Just wait until they turn two, the terrible twos! Their favorite word is "NO!" They don't even think before they utter that mighty "NO!" They are the "boss" at that stage of the game, and don't try to deny them that status!

I do not believe, however, that children should be awarded for bad behavior. They are certainly not cute when they are downright naughty and rude. I sometimes see parents on public television weeping bitterly because their seven and eight year old kids have become terrorists! Even the family pets seem to be in constant terror of them. Dad might be a six-footer and 200 pounds, but there he sits beside this little child with tears flowing down his face because he can't handle the situation! The viewing audience knows exactly how to fix little Johnnie once and for all in the few minutes of seeing his sweet little face on the television screen, but mommy and daddy don't have a clue what to do! "My little Johnnie slaps me, trashes my house, refuses to go to school, refuses to turn off the television and video games, and terrorizes his older brothers and sisters!"

Before you know it, Super Nanny or Dr. Phil is called to the rescue. I sometimes think to myself, "Just give little Johnnie to me for one or two days, and he would be fixed for life, free of charge!" I just love a challenge. I would not beat him, but he would certainly get the message. I strongly believe that children should have no problem identifying who is in charge in the home. They should be very clear on that because, believe me, if they get mixed messages or are confused as to the role of mom and dad, everyone will be in serious trouble. I never had that problem as a kid, neither did my siblings. Thank God, I never turned out too badly!

When little children burp or pass gas, they make no apologizes. If they sneeze, their little hands do not get in the way to stifle that sneeze, neither do they grab the Kleenex box. If they spit up or make a mess, they just go along with the flow.

Have you ever tried tasting a baby's formula? Just for fun, one day I poured a small amount of my niece's formula into my palm and tasted it. My, my, that stuff tasted like sawdust! As if I know what sawdust tastes like! But guess what, babies drink down that bland, tasteless food and do not complain. Later on in life, we introduce them to all sorts of junk. A candy bar here, sugar and salt there, and before you know it, they refuse to drink that formula anymore! They soon start demanding double servings of McDonald's and Wendy's and Dairy Queen.

When we see them ballooning right before our very eyes, then we ask this oft repeated question, "Where did I go wrong?" Surely they did not go grocery shopping for the family! Those empty calories were brought home by someone older than they! We sometimes create monsters that we are powerless to tame or kill. We have become a generation of "don't cook at home anymore, honey. Just call up a restaurant or fast food place, and we are ready to go."

There is so much that some of us stuffy, overly cultured adults can learn from these young ones. Children see food as something to sink their teeth into and have big fun of it. They take hold of it with their hands and into their mouths it goes. Who cares about a knife and fork? All ten fingers get the licking that they deserve after those children have eaten their fill. They know when they are full; then they turn off the engine! Have you ever tried giving a baby a bottle when it does not want it? That tongue becomes a bulldozer as it pushes that bottle away!

I love to see boys all dressed up in their smart little suits and girls in their ponytails and little pretty, lacey dresses. One songwriter said that the nearest thing to heaven is a child and that there's a special kind of sunshine in its smiles. I really understand what he meant. Most children are quite cute. Just by observing my nieces and nephews as well as my patients, I see lovable young folks. I believe that every person has within him or her the capability for greatness. We were born to become champions and deserve to become the best person we were destined to be. That's our right, and we should claim it every minute of every day that we live.

Let's shift gears a little and examine a baby's body. Take a good hard look at a baby's feet and especially its heels. Those heels seem to be as rounded as their knees! Those feet were not meant for walking, just for nibbling on! One day, out of the blue, this young person decides that he wants to take a step or two into the upright position and independently too! He gets the courage of ten, holds on to something like a chair, then he says to himself, "I have been practicing to move around on my hands and knees for a while now. I feel pretty comfortable doing so, but now I feel that it's time to do something exciting and different. I could be charged for speeding because I have been traveling quite a few miles per hour on all fours.

"For nine long months I was held captive in my mother's uterus surrounded by water. Mine was like a mini Hoover Dam or like the great flood of Noah's days. Granted, I kicked up a storm and fought an unholy war right there in my compartment, and they had to let me out, eventually. If you put me in that same quantity of water or even less and left me unattended then I would surely die by drowning and the judge and jury would later charge you with murder. Isn't life a mystery! I was living large, I tell you! I didn't even have to breathe on my own; life was good.

"Later I demanded that they cut the cord that bound me to my mother. 'What cord?' you might be asking. That umbilical cord of course! Now I request my freedom. No one is going to restrict or curtail my movement any longer, absolutely no one. I am going to walk!"

He makes his first step only to hit the hard floor. As he beholds stars and the nine planets, he puts this walking business on hold for a time! That temporary setback is only a steppingstone to try even harder. He is back to his four-wheel drive but only for a limited time. "I know I can, and I must," he thinks.

Okay, fellow, hold on to a chair again. Make a wide base with those short stubby legs, chin up, and chest forward. One, two, three ... go for it. "Yes, I did it! I took two steps. Three cheers for this pro. I know I am going to stumble and fall many times in the future. I am going to goof up, make poor judgments at times, but I am going to be okay. The race is not for the swift but to him who endures to the end!"

So this little child, over time, assumes the upright position using the "front wheel drive," and he soon becomes a pro. Heaven bless him! Who says that life is easy or was meant to be easy? Even the birthing process is not easy for both mother and baby. That baby was an active participant. He had to push his way out, and he would have been slapped on his buttocks if he didn't cry on his own. Crying is not such a bad thing after all. We all started our lives crying, but I hope that we don't go out the same way! We owe it to our children to have good memories of their growing up years and to keep wonderful traditions alive.

I have observed people through every stage of their lives. Through each phase we all say to some degree, "Look out world, here I come!" Every step of the way is new to us. We might see others go through that particular period, but we ourselves have never been there before. It is so amazing how quickly each phase changes. What a difference a few years make in the life of a child who we use to pick up, burp, and give piggyback rides to, and the next thing we know, it seems as if he is ready to go off to college! The teenage years with their possibilities as well as challenges are noteworthy times each of us goes through. Peer pressure on all sides, hormones jumping up and down in our bloodstream, and the quest to establish autonomy can leave some young persons wondering what on earth is happening to them! That is why they need wise positive input from those who have been there before.

Over the years I have looked to plenty of senor citizens for advice and support. Some of them are just so wise. My mother read a lot when she was younger and usually quoted famous writers who wrote such things as "Beautiful young people are accidents of nature, but beautiful old folks are works of art"; "It is magnificent to grow old, if one keeps young"; or "Never tell an old lady the truth, especially if she asks you for it!" Then she would add with a chuckle, "But there's no fool like an old fool!" Then my dad who was a soldier would say, "Old soldiers never die, they just fade away!"

Some seniors seem to take upon themselves the responsibility of becoming keepers of the past. They have to tell us what happened in what year and brief us on the "good old days" when a dollar went a far way and when their houses were left unlocked. They can remember what happened sixty years ago but can't remember where they last put their pair of spectacles even though it is sitting right there on the tip of their nose!

I sometimes compare and contrast them with children. Obviously, not one size fits all. Some live to be 110 and are mentally sharp as a brass tack, while others decline rapidly and regress to infantile or childlike behavior in their 80s. Some of them start asking the same questions again and again as do children. Their skin becomes very soft and smooth like a baby's. Some prefer to "gum" their food or have it pureed before they eat it than to wear dentures. They are prone to falls, so you will notice them holding on to objects and using a wide base when walking. Sometimes they lose control of their bladder and bowel and return to wearing diapers just like babies. They sometimes drool and need a bib. They have private conversations with themselves just as they did when they were children.

My mother is now a senior citizen in her own rights. She turned 100 on October 31, 2012. We planned a big party for her. She gets a little bit slower and more forgetful by the day but in the same breath more outspoken and very assertive. She used to handle the family's finances and knew quite well how to cut, stretch, and carve the meager earnings that my dad made. She was a great economist. Things improved drastically over the years for us, but her need to be in charge of the bank account has not.

One evening some years ago, just for fun, I gave her the helper's pay because she insisted that this was still her home, and "I am supposed to have money to pay everybody who works here!" I watched her from a safe distance putting the money where I was certain she would never remember. I marked the spot well. When it was time for the helper to go home for the weekend, I asked the million-dollar question, "Are you ready to pay the helper?" I still smile each time I remember her answer after tearing the place apart looking for the money she had hidden.

"Where do you expect me to get money from? Have you ever seen me leave this house even for one day to go to any job?" She has always been prim and very proper, so her defensive answer caught me off guard. I kindly showed her where she had hidden the money. Her response was, "I never put it there in the first place, so why are you showing it to me!" That was a no-win situation.

I usually spend most of my vacation time with my mom every year. I was just about to return home to New York when I told her something that I cannot remember right now. I am fast becoming a senior citizen myself—I can't remember a thing! Anyway, in a short space of time I asked her what I had said and she was unable to tell me. To my embarrassment, I remarked to her, "How could you have forgotten so quickly; I just told you a second ago."

She sarcastically said to me, "Pardon me, I have never been old before. This is new and very strange to me!" That statement was so profound and so true. All the way back on the airplane I thought of my mother's statement. "I have never been old before; this is new and strange to me." Before I retired to bed that night, I composed this poem with her in mind, and I later mailed a copy to her.

> "I Have Never Been Old Before"
> Please be patient with me
> When I fail to hear or see,
> Forget what you said a moment ago,
>
> Can't understand things *you* think I should know.
> You might never understand, my dear,
> The anxiety, dread, and fear
> I'm prone to face each passing day,

Wondering what to do or what to say.
You see, I've never been old before.
It's all brand new and strange to me; therefore,
Lend me your time and your ear

And show me that you really care.
I was once young and beautiful,
Wrinkle-free and graceful.
I could run, play, and dance.

Me, get tired? Not a chance!
Now I've entered my second childhood.
And like a new kid in the neighborhood,
It will take me some time to adjust

But I know I will and I must.
I can recall events of long ago
But not what happened a day or so.
I have to watch every step I take

For my own safety's sake.
I once could run the marathon;
Now I need someone to lean on.
When I take forever to finish my meal,

Believe me, it's a big deal!
Allow me some measure of independence,
Dignity, self-respect, and patience.
Patience with myself when I make a mess,

Knowing I'm still myself, nonetheless.
The person in the mirror, is it really me?
Where is the beauty I used to be?
The jet black hair and beauty spots

Are now replaced with silver and aged-spots.
But I feel just as lovely as ever.
I'll accept myself for who I really am and never
Be ungrateful for my many yesteryears,
Because I have been blessed in so many ways.

After I penned this poem, I thought of the lovely folks at the opposite end of the spectrum, the young. Childhood and teenage years call for added patience and tolerance on the part of adults in order for young folks to become well-adjusted individuals later in life. I sometimes reflect on times and circumstances that have helped to shape my life. There are things I wished I would have done differently or not done at all. I sometimes wish I could go back in time and erase all the negative comments, the slights, and the discouragements hurled at me as a child and youth.

Teachers exert a very strong influence on kids, and I have had my share of fortunetellers who looked into their invisible crystal balls and saw only failure for some of their students. On the other hand, there were those who sought to bring out the best in us, their students, and made sacrifices and invested time and energy into helping us become adults of whom they could be proud.

I have always been a self-proclaimed advocate for the less fortunate. I love children, and I get chills when I see them blossoming into young people determined to beat the odds and become great. I sometimes look back in time and actually thank the folks who never gave me one word of affirmation because they gave me weapons with which to fight. Shortly after I composed, "I Have Never Been Old Before," I decided to give the children and young adults their say, so I wrote the following poem.

"I Have Never Been Young Before"
This world is new and strange to me.
I have never been here before, so you see
I'll need some time to cope and adjust,
Learn how to survive and how to trust.

This spot in the universe called earth,
Has been my home since my birth.
I never asked to be born in the first place,
Or to be a member of the human race!

I came as an innocent little tot,
Sleeping, crying, and laughing a lot.
How I learn to do these things
Is still a mystery each day brings.

Who is this bright-eyed kid in the mirror,
Cute, cuddly, knowing nothing named sorrow?
It's me, wearing that big toothless grin,
Determined to make it in this world and win.

Be patient with me when I take my first step and fall;
I've never walked before at all.
Forgive me when I make a mess,
And keep on loving me nonetheless.

I've never been a child before.
I'm inexperienced, prone to err each hour.
Help me tie my lace, brush my teeth, comb my hair,
And reassure me that you'll always be there.

I was born free to choose my way
How to behave, what to do, and what to say.
Give me a chance to try something new
Even if I won't be half as good as you.

Allow me to fall and rise again
Make my own mistakes and try to gain
Wisdom and strength in the process
And with time become a great success.

If I mess up and make stupid decisions,
Kindly pardon my indiscretions.
I need your empathy and understanding
And that you'll be in my corner not withstanding.

Help me discover who I really am,
Anything else would be a total sham.
Leave a light in the window each night,
That would be enough to let me know that I might

Have a place called home
Wherever in this harsh world I might roam.

I'd then know being young once in my life
Was worth all the effort and the strife.

Chapter Thirteen

My Pact With God

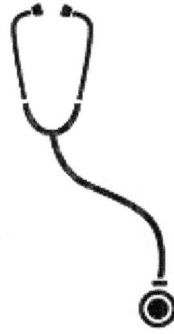

At the end of two years, my classmates and I were ready to write the qualifying examination as set by the Nursing Counsel of Jamaica. One Friday evening I got myself a sturdy cardboard box, put all my textbooks and notes in it, tied a string around it, and placed it in the back of my closet. I told myself that after two whole years of studying, a weekend of cramming would be a waste of time. If I had not gained enough knowledge to pass the examination, it was hopeless. I went to church over the weekend, prayed a special prayer for everyone who would be taking the exam that God would have His way in the outcome.

Each of us was given an envelope on which to write our name and address so that the results of the exam could be mailed to us. Monday morning dawned clear and bright. It felt good to be alive. As was my custom since childhood, I prayed, read my Bible, and thanked God for His leadership in my life up unto that point.

I got dressed, but just before I left the house, I went back to my bedroom, knelt down beside my bed, and made a pact with God. This was one bold undertaking, but I felt very confident that the God who had started me down this path would be more that capable of helping me to complete it! I asked God, my Jehovah-jireh, to grant me a sense of calmness and serenity and bring back to my memory and that of my classmates the things we had learned during our studies. I then asked God one very special favor.

I said, "Dear Father, You know the desire of my heart, a desire that goes back as far as I can remember. Now, I am just a few hours from actualizing that dream and desire. However, if in Your knowledge, You see that I, in the future, would not be a caring, compassionate nurse and that I would not treat the folks You love as dearly as You love me well, then don't allow me to pass this examination, Amen!"

I got up from my knees with a peace that was very hard to describe. Incidentally, on Sunday night while I was sleeping, I had a dream, and in that dream I saw every question that appeared on the examination! Those were not the days of multiple-choice questions or computerized tests. We had to write essay type answers.

After the exam we were given two weeks vacation time. I left the city and headed to the place I loved best, my home on the farm. My dad was a farmer, a "tiller of the soil." I still go home quite often because I don't want to miss my way or forget my roots. At that time it was mango season. I ate mangoes to my heart's content. I had the pleasure of walking from one end of my parents' farm to the other and visiting places I had once played at as a child. I had a chance to relive, for a short time, childhood passions such as kicking off my shoes and running through rain puddles and smelling the earth after it rained. That aroma has got to be Mother Nature's ultimate air freshener! I saw stars in the night sky, heard crickets chirping, and saw fireflies darting here and there!

All too quickly, the two weeks expired, and I had to go back to face the real world. Within a short time Mr. Postman made his presence known as he delivered the day's mail. Among the stack of mail was one with a very familiar handwriting that seemed to say, "Herein lies thy fate!" For one second my heart skipped a beat or two.

I handed the envelope containing the news of my future to my sister's helper and ran to the safety of the bathroom. Within a short space of time, she was knocking on the door and yelling, "Come out, come out; you passed, you passed!"

This was music to my ears. I took the letter this time not with trembling hands but with confidence because I know that my God is an awesome God!

"The pleasure is ours to inform you ..."

That was enough pleasure as far as I was concerned. I had no need to finish the letter at that time.

The pact I had made with God would have been futile if God was not there to nudge me and remind me of who I was and what I was capable of becoming and that if I became self-sufficient, haughty, and arrogant then I would fall flat on my face. I have been holding tightly to God since I was a child—I grew up with Him! I am cognizant that I am like an animal born in captivity and that I am incapable of fending for myself successfully without Him.

Now that I had passed the qualifying examination, I was ready to complete a yearlong internship in the clinical areas I had covered over the previous two years of my training. I was given the title of "nurse intern."

My group was divided into two. One group was sent to an area where tourists frequent, and the other remained in Kingston. It seemed unreal as to the rapidity at which that year passed. I grew up fast that year. I survived night shifts, the emergency room, the operating room, medical/surgical nursing, and all the other areas we were assigned. One Friday evening I assisted a doctor in the ER, and all we did from the start of the shift to its close was suture up human hides! Casualties of every sort were brought in. I saw emergency room nurses making split-second decisions that impacted life or death, and I wondered if I would be capable of doing so in the future. Time had convinced me that all things were possible if I put my trust in God.

Chapter Fourteen

Graduation

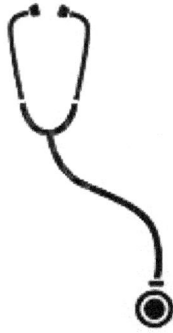

My dream was not just a dream anymore; it had become a physical reality.

My father was the only one in my family who really encouraged my dream. I knew that my mother and my siblings cared about me and loved me and wanted what was best for me. Their concern was that I might not have had the stamina to do nursing. Why not go into teaching and enjoy the long vacation periods, have all weekends off, and be able to sleep in a warm comfortable bed every night? Who wants to clean and dress those big smelly ulcers? Who in their right mind would want to stick people with needles?

Well, I am sure they knew me well enough to realize I knew exactly what I wanted. I could be very appreciative of their wise council, but I was determined to have my way, the way planned out for me by God.

Graduation day came at last. I was given a piece of paper with my name affixed to it, stating that I was qualified to be a member of the healthcare profession with all the rights and privileges of Florence Nightingale herself! I had within my hands the care of my patients. God has the ultimate power of life, but I am an instrument He uses to accomplish His biddings. I asked Him, amid the activity of that evening, to help me every day to strive for excellence, listen to His still small voice when He speaks clearly and distinctly, and leave the rest to Him.

I exchanged my blue and white uniform to don another. This time, the one I had longed to wear since childhood, an immaculate white one. I held my head high and humbly acknowledged the presence of my kinfolks who conceded after they knew I had won the trophy of a lifetime

As I sat there in that crowded auditorium that graduation day, my mind raced back to the first time I had seen a real patient in a real bed in a real hospital.

I also thought of that nurse, my angel in human form. Was she still alive? Was she a real human being? My dad and my siblings just could not remember seeing her again. We have heard of angels being sent on special missions to earthlings, and I wondered if she was one of those! If I had had the pleasure of having her there beside me during that graduation exercise, what would I have said to her? Maybe, I would have been silent, but that silence would have been louder that any spoken word.

Chapter Fifteen

My First Job as a Registered Nurse

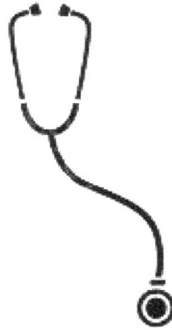

After I graduated I took a whole month off to mentally and physically gear myself up for the road ahead. During that time my mother and I planted several beds of roses and revived some of her old plants as well. Rest is said to be a change of occupation, so I certainly rested during that month. All too soon I knew it was time to start practicing nursing, earning some real money, and growing up!

I made the decision to go back to the very hospital in which I had been inspired to become a nurse. In fact, I worked on the very floor on which my father had been a patient.

My very first day on the job as a registered nurse is an experience I will never forget. A soon to be retired nurse was assigned to be my preceptor. When I was introduced to her, even though she knew me since my birth, she at that time had no clue as to who I really was! She must have wondered who this young upstart was just standing there and smiling! My voice and features finally convinced her that I was, indeed, the long-legged kid who used to run through the hospital's long corridor as a shortcut to get to and from school.

She was quite thrilled to "show me the ropes," and I grasped the ropes in a relatively short period of time. The folks with whom I had grown up were very happy to have one of their own coming back to take care of them. Before long I *graduated* from my preceptor and was ready to launch out on my own. It posed a bit of a challenge to do the rotating shifts at first. I had to change from day to evening then to night shift, but I survived.

I, at times, was a bit insecure. I did not have my tutors to rely on or hide behind if I erred. I was on my own. I had a bit of withdrawal after being dependent on them for so long. In those moments I reminded myself that I had the best Person, the best Preceptor in my corner. I had the Greatest Physician who would be more than willing to show me the ropes any time and during any shift, so I had nothing to be perturbed about.

As I adjusted to my new job, I remembered a lesson my father had taught me about driving. My father had a British made green Austin Cambridge car. That car was built to last a lifetime. It boasted real steel and iron, and I am quite sure that if any modern day automobile should have collided with it, that new model would have been totaled!

Nothing on that car was semi or automatic—stick shift, clutch, etc. After driving a few miles, I needed no further exercise for the day. I had a good workout! The steering wheel was very tough and Papa would say to me, "Don't fight that steering wheel, just push and draw, push and draw. Pretend that this steering wheel is the face of a clock. Place your hands on it as if it were quarter to three. Just push to the right then the left, push and draw, push and draw! Don't put too much muscle into the auto, my child, just learn to keep the car on the road! What did I say? Just learn to keep the car on the road!" We laughed and had fun while keeping the car on the road!

I translated my father's "Learn to keep the car on the road" to my new job: Learn the hospital's routine and get familiar with the everyday happenings, the policies and procedures, and not aim to be the hospital's matron or CEO! When I got that message then I became more confident with each passing day.

Chapter Sixteen

My First Blood Transfusion

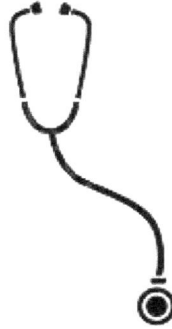

Shortly after my training wheels were off and I was on my own, I began the afternoon shift. One day I got a call from the emergency room that a patient who was having some gastro-intestinal bleeding was being transferred to my ward and that he needed a blood transfusion as soon as possible. The patient arrived on the floor shortly thereafter with intravenous fluid in progress. I observed that the patient's intravenous site was red and swollen.

It so happened that the patient in question was my father's best friend who had not seen me in many years neither did he know I was a nurse. His first reaction was that of pride as well as surprise! I orientated him to his new environment and informed him of his need to be transfused. Everything seemed to be going okay, but guess what? The needle in his arm needed to be removed and put in another spot! I had never inserted a needle in anybody's vein before. I was familiar with the principle and had observed it being done on several occasions, but seeing and doing are worlds apart.

I thought of making an emergency exit, so I didn't have to deal with the situation. In fact, the road behind the hospital led straight to my house! Then I thought to myself, *What's the worst thing that can happen right now?*

My pride was at stake. Big deal! So what? I was the newest member of staff. There were always resource people around, so why worry?

I guess that when we are young we all have something to prove to somebody. We have to prove to our parents that we are responsible, so we work hard to gain their trust. We have to prove to our teachers that we are good students by getting good grades and passing their examinations. Then we spend a good part of our lives studying to start a career. Later we land ourselves a job. A probationary period is given for us to prove to the powers that be that we know what we are doing, and we cannot afford to mess up. When we think we have had enough practice on keeping a car on the road, and we believe that it's time to go for our driver's license, we have to prove to the person who has the power to give you that piece of paper, that the most important part of the car is you, the "nut behind the steering wheel!", as I once saw in a magazine. Is this ego, good judgment, or just survival instinct?

Now that I am older and I believe wiser, I have very little left to prove to anybody! On the other side of the coin, some folks don't care what others think of them. They just do what pleases them. At the end of the day, I wonder who is less stressed? Anyway, let me get back to that needle that was supposed to be put into my patient's vein! This was the ultimate litmus test to prove to my father's friend that I was no dummy but a real nurse.

I had to have an emergency conference call with my Consultant. I assisted my patient into bed and made him comfortable, and when the nurses' assistant began to take his vital signs, I took off to the bathroom. I said, "Look, God, I have never done this before on my own. I need Your help, and I need it stat. Thanks for answering me. Amen."

I emerged from that bathroom with an inexpressible peace and calm. I assembled all the stuff I needed to do the procedure, explained to the patient what I was going to do, and then I started. I tied a tourniquet around the gentleman's arm, and the biggest, juiciest vein appeared. Even a blind nurse could have seen that vein! That port of entry was a nurse's dream! One shot and the needle glided with precision into that vein! I connected the intravenous tubing to the patient's needle and then later began giving him a liter of fluid. I took a brief timeout to return to the safety of the bathroom to say a quick but big "thank you" to my Consultant, God.

The next step, the blood transfusion, seemed easier even though I had never done it before on my own. The needle was still hanging in there, so I just needed someone to verify that I was giving the right blood to the right patient. My dad's friend got his two units of blood. He didn't have any adverse reaction, and no further bleeding occurred. By the following morning he was discharged. He could not wait to see my father to brag about me. Was it beginner's luck that saved the day? I don't think so. I believe it was by divine intervention.

Nursing, as I was told as a student nurse, is an art and a science, and I have added to that statement copious amounts of commonsense. I acquired a lot of practical skills using commonsense and knowledge during the two years and six months I worked at my first job. I grew to love the staff and patients, some I had grown up with and others I met along the way. Some patients are just unforgettable both in negative as well as positives ways.

For example, one night when I reported for my shift one of the doctors who was attending to a very sick patient began telling me how busy he had been all day and that he needed to go home and get some rest. He had been trying for a long time to find a vein to give this patient intravenous fluids, and he could not get any access. He reassured me that if I really needed help during the night shift, I should feel free to contact the on-call doctor. This incidence took place approximately four months after I graduated. A brief report was given to me at the change of shift. The nurse giving me the report was very concerned for the patient of this doctor.

The patient was admitted during the evening shift with temperatures well over 103 degrees along with diarrhea and vomiting. He was a teenager and had a very life-threatening gastro-intestinal disease. I had never cared for any patient with that diagnosis; I had only read about it during my training. All I knew was that I was dealing with a very sick young man and that his life hung in a balance. I don't believe that the doctor knew how ill the child really was or he wouldn't have run off and left me to fend for myself.

The patient was so dehydrated that his eyes seemed to be receding and his skin was very dry and warm to the touch. When I checked his temperature at that time, it was 104 degrees! He became quite delirious. His speech was incoherent, and he became restless, so I had to put up side rails to prevent him from falling off the bed. I thought about my father's wise counsel, "Learn to keep the car on the road!" I translated that into,

"Milicent, set priorities, set priorities! What is the most important thing for this patient now?"

So I made sure he was safe. Next I determined we needed to reduce his temperature as quickly as possible. I had to become cruel in order to be kind, so I instructed the nurses' aide to get ice and literally pack it all over his body. To my horror and dismay, the patient began passing frank bloody diarrhea. That was double jeopardy. That child needed intravenous fluids and a blood transfusion stat.

The ward was dimly lit, so I knew it would be difficult to find a vein to start any form of hydration on this very ill child. As a matter of fact, the doctor had made several attempts to start an IV without success. But there was no way I was going to stand there and let this child die! There was a desk lamp on the ward with a mind of its own. Depending on its mood, it would give some light for a limited time and then just turn itself off! I asked the aide to plug the lamp in next to the patient's bedside. At first she assured me that that was a waste of time because of the lamp's history and disposition! I knew that the lamp would work because it had to work! No other choice was offered to it!

The lamp was turned on, and God allowed it to give off enough light for me to find a very big vein. I got it on the very first attempt. The patient was given intravenous fluids and a blood transfusion during the night and by morning his temperature returned to normal and the bleeding never recurred. Within a week he was discharged from the hospital. Close to a year later he came back to see me. What a difference a year made! It was such a joy to see him again.

For a little under three years I worked at that hospital, and I really had a good time. Supplies were not in abundance—we had to improvise sometimes without compromising patient safety, but we made do. Our patients respected us as healthcare professionals and were grateful to us for whatever care they received. People were not quick to sue for whatever reason. Lack of insurance was never an issue in receiving care both in our clinics and hospitals. Nurses had time for their patients and life was less stressful then. But an opportunity of a lifetime was offered to me, and I did not refuse it. I immigrated to Canada, but I took with me the same old fundamentals of nursing to pilot me on my new adventure.

Chapter Seventeen

Oncology Nursing

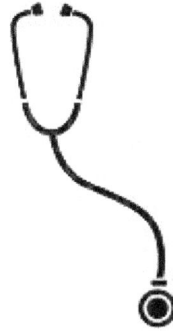

Some of the wonderful things about the nursing profession are its universal practices and that we speak the same language be it French, English, Spanish, or Dutch. That sameness all stems from its fundamentals and principles. Methods of doing procedures might vary from one institution to another or even from one country to the next, but the principles of knowing and doing those things are very similar.

When I arrived in a beautiful city in the province of Alberta, it seemed I was in Utopia at its best, and I was determined to blend into that perfect state. I arrived in the summertime with a dry weather totally different from that which I had experienced all my life. I touched down amid oilfields. On other occasions I had landed close to oceans, seas, and rivers; now I was landing in oilfields! That was a rich environment! When I think of Alberta, many things come to mind: chinook winds, the majestic Rocky Mountains as old as time itself, Banff National Park, Lake Louise, and Columbia Icefields with glaciers many centuries old and thick. The famous Calgary Stampede was then in full swing. That is, indeed, the ultimate rodeo. Natives and visitors become instant cowboys and cowgirls, donning jeans, cowboy hats, and boots. I was caught up in the spirit of the old west.

I enjoyed a few weeks of vacation time, but ultimately I realized I needed a job in order to survive. In a short time I was offered a position in one of the city's Provincial Hospitals. This was a far cry from the one I had worked at back home. One of the familiar words I had heard during my training and in my previous hospital was improvise. We improvised without compromising patient safety, but in this hospital, improvising was next to blasphemy. I was like a child in a candy store wondering which of the goodies to select.

My very first day on the job began with a twelve-hour shift, twelve long hours! The plus that those long shifts had was that the days off were just splendid! I received a brief orientation to the very important places such as the morgue, pharmacy, emergency room, and cafeteria. There was no one to precept me to the routine of the place, its equipment, or anything. I saw machines and equipment that were unfamiliar to me, but I was not overly perturbed because I was confident that my Consultant would be there for me. I didn't leave Him behind because I knew I couldn't make too many decisions independently without botching things up.

I must confess that at first I felt a few butterflies fluttering in my stomach, and if the climate was not cool that time of year, I would have sweated a bit. I was given a godsend nurse, Sue, who adopted me. I never asked for help, but for some unexplained reason, she volunteered to show me the ropes. Her days off seemed to coincide with mine, and in a short space of time I was familiar with the medications, equipment, and the routine of the unit. Before long, I graduated from Sue with flying colors! Thanks to my buddy.

I remained on that floor for about six months. One day, out of the blue, I was informed that the head nurse for the soon to be opened Oncology Unit and the other nurse coordinators wanted to meet with me. My heart skipped several beats. Was I being given the boot? My probationary period was over, what next?

After the usual small talk and formalities, I was told that I had been handpicked to join the staff of the new Oncology Unit that would be up and running within a month or even earlier. "If you need time to think it over, I will wait, but I really believe you should accept this offer. It's a brand new world, and I am sure you will like it," said my head nurse. First of all, I was totally unfamiliar with oncology; I had no clue as to what to expect except that it had to do with cancer treatment. There I was looking quite intelligent with an air of enthusiasm as if I really knew what I was getting into.

As if by sheer reflex, I spoke with conviction in a voice that was not too familiar to my ears. It sounded like I was listening to a very interesting conversation and wondering, *Who is that person? I'd really like to meet her!*

"I would love to be a part of this unit, and I am sure I will be a good team player," I said. Team player? Who was I fooling?

Well, the panel seemed quite pleased with my decision, but the team player had some serious contemplation to do! The die was cast, and I decided to step up to the plate, maintain that "intelligent" look, and prove my strength of character. I had nothing to lose, and it seemed I had the prospect of gaining a lot. Eight nurses were hired to open that unit. We implemented new policies and procedures relevant to oncology and got our supplies in order. We were oncology nurses in training for one of the most challenging but rewarding specialties in nursing.

Oncology is basically the study and treatment of tumors. An oncologist and oncology nurses' primary concern and interest is cancer prevention and treatment. The American Cancer Society defines cancer as, "A group of diseases characterized by uncontrolled growth and spread of abnormal cells." Ours is a specialty that requires a great deal of emotional stability, empathy, and listening skills. I hate cancer in all its forms. To me, it is evil—totally unnecessary, selfish, mean, and heartless—and its only purpose is to disrupt life and living. As specialists in the field, we dedicate our time and energy to giving our patients a fighting chance through education, chemotherapy, radiotherapy, pain management, nutrition, and supportive therapy, and when all else fails, we make ourselves available to them to the very end.

Sue, my buddy I mentioned before, was also a part of the team. We were the first two nurses to officially open the unit. That opening night was the longest night of my entire life! We had one self-caring patient who was not even supposed to have been there in the first place. He had come to receive radiotherapy, but because of the long distance from his home and icy road conditions, he had been offered a bed for the night. Sue and I took turns checking on our sleeping "patient" all night. The heating system was not even functioning well, so we got portable heaters and kept our winter coats on so we would not be found frozen to death when the morning staff came on! We had a deadline to meet in opening that unit even if we did not have any patients. During the shift, Sue and I put charts together, labeled cabinets, and by and large found things to do to kill the time.

This unit was built with patient comfort in mind. It is a multimillion-dollar state of art structure equipped with all the luxury of a hotel. Patients were encouraged to wear their casual clothes and enjoy the beautiful things that the place had to offer. We had patients who had lost their hair to chemotherapy walking around without hats or wigs, and they were not self-conscious about it. As our patient population increased so did the staff. It was so gratifying to see survivors and their families returning every once in a while just to visit. Over the years our unit treated sports celebrities, some who climbed noteworthy mountains; best-selling authors; and some folks in the movie industry.

I am so humbly proud to have had a hand in the history of that great work environment. I learned a lot, and my big gamble paid big dividends. I love oncology very much even though at times it gets tough to watch people who you have grown to love simply fade before our very eyes. We just have to pick up the pieces and move forward, hoping that one day we will find a cure for this monster.

During my time there I met and took care of some patients who became my inspiration. Many a time when I decided to throw a lavish pity party for myself with all the melancholy guests—"Why me, why not some-one else?" "Poor me." "Why can't I be happy like my friends?"—I canceled it and drew strength from those folks who had so much unfavorable things hurled at them but managed to keep a stiff upper lip. There was one young lady in particular who made me love her even though I fought with claws and determination not to get attached to her or any other patient for that matter. There are some folks who just seem to work their way into our lives and take up residence there, and we cannot do otherwise but give to them the key and privilege to stay as long as they want!

This young lady I just mentioned was diagnosed with cancer while in her early twenties. By that time, the cancer had spread throughout her body. Her bones were like eggshells. Ever so often she would have a pathological fracture, mostly to her spine. When I met her she had shrunken a great deal. She looked like an old woman in a young adult's body, all stooped and bent. We had to be especially careful when she was lifted or turned because her brittle bones would just snap.

She was in pain for most of her waking hours, but she fought back the tears with smiles as big as the full moon over the prairies. Avoidance is one of my coping mechanisms. I don't make it a habit of using it often, but it gives me a bit of time to plan my next move. In this patient's case, that action was near impossible. Even on my days off I found myself calling to find out how she was doing, and she knew exactly what days I would be back.

This patient had the warmest smile to brighten many a Canadian dreary winter month, and believe me, those months could be bone chillingly cold! She would inquire if I had arrived on the unit because she always seemed to have the need to tell me all that had transpired during my absence. Did I really need to hear? That seemed to be the highlight of her day, so why deprive her of that thrill? She read a lot and would give me a summery of her books, somewhat like a book report. Most times I had to remind myself that I had other patients to take care of. In those good old days, we had more staffing, so we had more time to spend one-on-one with patients and their families.

She went through yet another round of chemotherapy. After a while she began calling me Mom even though I was not much older than she was! Regardless of how strong we consider ourselves to be physically, emotionally or otherwise, this human machinery has an expiration date. Parts wear out, systems shut down, some can be repaired or replaced while others have just the manufacturer's lifetime warranty. Wear and tear, chemicals and lifestyle sometimes trigger our immune system to say, "Hold it; I've had enough, time to go."

Her time was winding down rapidly, but who would be brave enough to notify her aged parents? You see, this young lady was born to parents who had practically given up hopes of having a child. We have authority over a lot of things in life, but we have none over a child that refuses to be conceived! Then this precious gift was given to them. She was the apple of their eye, and their love for her went without question. Now they were losing her to cancer and eventually to death itself. Time was of the essence, so her parents were called. They lived on a farm outside of the city, and on that cold icy afternoon, in their desire to see their child alive for what was probably the very last time, the father lost control of the vehicle and it overturned, killing both parents instantly.

We are powerless to explain certain things that happen in our personal lives and in the lives of others. Even Christians struggle with the notion of a just God who allows bad things to happen to good people. This is where I believe faith in God means everything. Some folks console themselves by believing that they go to heaven instantly when they die. That gives them strength to carry on. I don't personally subscribe to that notion, but I do believe that one day we will see the folks we loved best when Jesus returns to take us home. It takes a lot of faith in God to hold on to things that appear to make absolutely no sense at all, but we have to understand that faith cannot be explained by logical reasoning!

I was not at work on the day when the accident occurred and my patient was dying. Thank God I was not there because I do not believe I could have handled the situation well. She was by then slipping in and out of consciousness. When the tragic news finally reached the unit, the priest was called to break the news to the patient. I can only imagine what was racing through her mind when that priest took up his position at her bedside. Was he there to let her know that she had just a limited time left? Did he want to offer her some sort of consolation to buoy her spirits? The suspense was short-circuited as he gave it to her straight. "Your parents will not be coming to see you today. They were killed this afternoon in an accident."

This brave heart responded with a smile and, in a voice as beautiful as she herself was, said, "That's okay, we will die together." She was not angry; the loss of her parents and the suffering she had endured for such a long time eclipsed into nothingness. She was ready to go. Within a short period of time she took her last breath and peacefully fell asleep. I missed her smiles, her wanting to know how my days off were, what plans I had for her for that day, and when I thought she would be going home. It seemed to be her all-consuming desire to know when she would be discharged. After what transpired, I made a pledge to never get attached to another patient, but I have broken that pledge often, and I still do.

I went full speed ahead in soaking up all I could get about oncology nursing. We had then began radium implant, immunotherapy, radiotherapy, and bone marrow transplants. We were growing by leaps and bonds, and progress was being made before our very eyes. We had a staff of doctors and nurses whose nationalities spanned the globe. We were like members of the United Nations, but we worked well together. Each of us brought something to the table, be it cultural belief, food, or skills. Each person felt important.

I believe that things happen in our lives to teach us important lessons and that some things are beyond our control. We find ourselves living in places where we never planned and doing stuff that was not on our "to do" list. I never had any plans to live in the United States of America and New York in particular. I had planned to live in Canada to a ripe old age. But I have been in New York for more than two decades, and I'm still contemplating my next move.

New York City is home to Lady Liberty; the George Washington Bridge, which spans the great divides between towns, boroughs, and states; Yankee Stadium; Radio City Music Hall; Madison Square Gardens; Central Park; Grand Central Station; the Brooklyn Bridge, and of course the United Nations building—all of these landmarks attest to the city's fame and status on the world map. The United Nations building draw heads of states together to make pertinent decisions to improve the world, but their efforts are like oil mixed with water, metal with clay. I, for the first time in my life, saw trains and boats and planes taking restless, weary travelers all over the place. I wondered at first if I could ever adjust to this state of confusion.

I must confess that my first visit gave me quite a culture shock. I had just left quiet, reserved, clean Alberta where pedestrians waited patiently for the traffic lights to change, regardless of the season, before attempting to cross the street. Then suddenly I saw literally hundreds of folks moving with the speed of light hurrying to who knows where. I said to myself, *This is madness!* This was like a jungle where survival seemed to be high on everyone's agenda. Could I survive? I guess time has told me that I, indeed, have in me the tenacity to do anything I put my mind to do with God's help.

"Rolling stone gathers no moss," I learned in school, but this rolling stone was determined to gather moss, gold, diamonds, knowledge, or whatever happened to come my way! I sing this song and I love it dearly:

> "This is my Father's world
> And to my listening ears
> All nature sings and round me rings
> The music of the spheres.
> This is my Father's world,
> Why should my heart be sad?
> The Lord is King,
> Let the heavens ring
> God reigns let the earth be glad."

This song sustains me when I feel overwhelmed or anxious because I am cognizant of the fact that this is my Father's world; therefore, I am special.

In this great metropolis I have found a mosaic not of colorful stones, glass, tile, or even wood but of people represented from every corner of the globe, each contributing to the whole to form a beautiful picture. You either love or leave New York. After living here for a long time, I have not given myself a chance to explore all that it has to offer. One day before I'm old, very old, I will savor its glory and might even write about it!

On my third visit to New York City, I decided to pull up roots from Canada and replant them in the States. I got myself a job after I was actually recruited by the institution. My specialty and skills were needed, and after a brief period of orientation, I was on my own. My love for my oncology patients has not diminished one bit since I first took care of my independent patient that cold opening night. Oncology has taught me the sad truth that life is fleeting and fragile, and it is not always a just taskmaster. We do not always get what we bargain for. It also has taught me that life is a priceless commodity from God to be treasured dearly and to be lived to the fullest. We need to live our grandest lives today because tomorrow is promised to nobody. Cancer, I observe, is no respecter of persons, class, caste, age, or status. It strikes sometimes without warning and puts many things on hold.

I have observed over the years that patients who have a strong support system through family, church affiliation, friends and who will themselves to survive usually make better strides over those who give up easily. A positive upbeat attitude makes a world of difference. The incidence of cancer is on the rise. Have we made many significant strides in the field of oncology? Yes, I think we have. One of the most important things I personally do for my patients is simply being there for them. Sometimes silence speaks more loudly than a pep talk and "I understand how you feel." No person understands how a person diagnosed with cancer feels save she who is diagnosed! Sometimes just the visible presence of another human being, holding a hand, a shoulder on which to lean, or a heart that tries to understand is all that a patient needs. My constant watchword is, "Here is your call bell. Use it when you need me; I'll be here!"

Chapter Eighteen

Memories Are Made of These

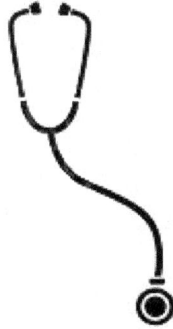

If I should go back in time and retrieve the most noteworthy and significant memories of my nursing career so far, I wonder which ones they would be. It would be quite difficult to do that, so I will now go into my library of memories and pull out a few of my very best from a shelf I label "Very Special." These very special encounters with the past do not necessarily mean that they were always filled with moonlight and roses or would they be the ones I would brag about while having a meal with folks who do not do what we nurses do! The not so pleasant experiences have served to make me a stronger and better person over the years.

Some of these incidences sound a little stranger than fiction. I am going to make a very conscious effort to omit names, places, and diagnoses, but if for any reason, these stories are familiar to anyone, my intention is not to cause grief or unpleasantness to anybody but rather to highlight the humanness of nursing. *Nursing is real!* These stories are authentic and honest, but they are not intended to reveal any patient or co-worker's personal and confidential information.

Henry Wadsworth Longfellow once wrote: "Look not mournfully into the past. It comes not back again. Wisely improve the present. It is thine. Go forth to meet the shadowy future, without fear, and with a manly heart."

I invite you now to fasten your seatbelts and come with me on a time odyssey—three decade and counting! As I travel down memory lane during my nursing career there have been things that I would have rather not seen or experienced, but this is the reality of it. Nursing is real. It's nothing like what is depicted on General Hospital, Grey's Anatomy, or ER, or some other type of television drama. As a matter of fact, I don't spend too much time watching them. I take my job seriously and my patients' lives are of paramount importance. And the following stories are from my years in the field. This is a whole saga all its own; this is NURSING!

My Father Loves Me!

I saw pictures of her before she was reduced to mere skin and bones. She was the type of woman who would have made Betty Davis seem like Plain Jane. Her eyes, flawless skin, and smiles said she loved life and embraced it in her own way until she was diagnosed with one of the world's most dreaded diseases with all the stigmas attached to it. Well, she was the "black sheep" in the midst of a family of religious zealots and how dare her disgrace this upright, spotless clan!

In spite of all that transpired, she still had support from her mom who visited her every chance she could, and I believe those visits were the highlight of my patient's day. Occasionally other family members would drop by for brief periods. I was assigned to her care when she was first admitted, and she was hell-bent on hurling all her pent-up anger and frustration at me for most of my shift. I refused to take her behavior as a personal attack, but at the same time I set limits for her and for myself. Anyway, over time I purposefully began chipping away at that tough, macho-type personality until I discovered a soft little heart beating there. I celebrated the moment when I got my first faint smile from her, and I lived in heightened expectancy that more were on the way.

As the days went by, she would give me glimpses into her life, her family, school, her father's high expectations of her, and the ultimate disease that had so eroded her entire being. I often wondered what was passing through this self-righteous father's mind. Did his wife give him a daily update or report of his daughter's worsening condition, and if she did, how did he respond? It seemed obvious that the end was very close for my patient, so I asked her if she wished me to contact her family, and she answered in the affirmative. She was dying, but her dad was on her mind.

"I wish above everything else to see my father and to know that he still loves me and is willing to forgive me. Then and only then will I know I am ready to die. Right now I am not sure I am ready."

I got the father's phone number and made a personal call to him. I identified who I was, told him that his child was very ill, and requested to see him. There was silence at the other end of the telephone. I continued to converse with a person who I had never met.

"Your daughter needs you, sir, and if you believe in what you preach, then you had better put it into action. She is very ill and asks for your forgiveness, forgiveness for what I do not know."

I guess that at that point I got a bit carried away, but I thought I was compelled to finish this mission, so I pressed on. "And let me tell you something else; if you cannot forgive your sick daughter, neither will God forgive you!" I gently hung up the phone.

He must have driven through all the red lights or had gotten every green one because in a relatively short time he presented himself on the unit and asked for me by name. My heart skipped several beats because I honestly felt I might have come on a little strong and that he might have decided to retaliate. That was not to be the case. He just wanted to see his child. I'm sure he never bargained for what he was facing. Could this be his beautiful daughter lying there in that bed? I felt his pain, but I decided to give him space and privacy.

He motioned to me to stay with him for a while. He was visibly shaken as he held his daughter ever so gently and tenderly in his arms for the last time. In those few brief moments, recollection of the past thirty years must have fast-forwarded through his mind. I imagined him recalling her taking her first step and falling, then scooping her up in his arms, brushing her knees and drying her tears. The times when he rocked her to sleep, cooled her feverish brow as she battled childhood illnesses, watched her tie her shoelaces and learn to ride a bike, watched her get all dolled up for her high school prom and later walked her down the aisle, a picture a loveliness, to exchange wedding vows. He just held her as he tried to stifle sobs that rocked his body. I cried not for myself but for them. Then I gave them privacy. There was bonding and closure and peace.

When he left, she called me in and said, "My father loves me, he told me so."

She had the smile of a winner. She was losing her life, but she had won the trophy of a lifetime—her father's forgiveness and love. Toward the end of the shift, she passed away peacefully as if she was touched by an angel.

That night before I retired to my bed, I called my dad and told him good night one more time and that I loved him dearly. I wanted to hear his voice and that was good enough for me.

I Can See, I Can See!

She was a ninety-plus-year-old great,-great-grandma who was a rare, precious treasure to her family. She was like a well-written history book to be read by generations to come. She held in her hand the unwritten pages of her family's lives, and I am sure that this great-great-grandma got a kick out of recalling and dramatizing stories of days of yore. Every day she would be visited by her kinfolks who would spend time fussing over her and making sure her needs were met.

Her admission to the hospital was nothing out of the ordinary, just an age-related illness. Great-great-grandma's condition improved, and toward the end of her stay someone came up with the most brilliant idea. You see, for the past ten years of her life, she had lost her vision in both eyes, but her sense of hearing was as sharp as ever. In my sometimes pensive mood, I once in a while ask myself, if for some strange reason I was told I had to give up one of my senses completely, which would I opt to lose? Giving up my sense of sight would definitely be out of the question. No siree, don't even think about it! Do not dare touch my eyeballs!

I am a lover of nature and all the wonderful things that she has to offer. No one can describe colors to a blind person. How does one relate to another the awe of seeing winter budding into springtime, the beauty of sunrise and sunset, the winsome smiles of innocent children? I really believe God has a good sense of humor. The seemingly little things in nature still baffle some of the greatest minds in the scientific world, but to God they are just small stuff! He sees the lighter side of things. I was blessed to have lived on a farm in the countryside as a child. I had the freedom and time to see God's handiwork displayed lavishly every day. I often wondered how the spiders managed to spin such dainty yet strong and exquisite webs that can be found in the grandest palaces as well as lonely huts in the woods. Would those spiders ever run out of their silken material? The fireflies would be seen darting away as soon as darkness set in. Would they ever collide, and did they have built-in batteries or GPS? I often asked myself these questions. When I see flashes of lightening and stars in clusters on cloudless nights, I still stand amazed. I cannot but exclaim with the songwriter, "O Lord my God, how wonderful Thou art!"

What could I give in exchange for memories of seeing for myself places I once thought only existed in fairy tales, history books, or the Holy Bible? I have looked skyward into the face of the mighty Sphinx, walked into the largest pyramid of Egypt, and crossed the Nile River. I viewed treasures of King Tut enough to fill a whole floor of the great Egyptian museum. That boy was loaded! He was buried in solid gold caskets and with all the things needed to live it up big time in the afterlife!

I climbed the heights of Masada, stepped on the shores of the Dead Sea, 1,288 feet beneath sea level, and visited the site of the ancient Sodom and Gomorrah. I saw and walked in the Jordon River. I followed in the footsteps of Jesus as I walked the Via Dolorosa, the traditional way of the cross to the church of the Holy Sepulchre. I beheld Jesus' tomb in the Garden Tomb, believed to be the traditional site of Golgotha. I looked from my room in The Seven Arches Hotel atop the Mount of Olives and viewed the city of Jerusalem on cloudless nights. I saw the Sea of Galilee in her majestic splendor from the patio of the Jordan River hotel on a moonlit night and sailed on those ancient waters! I stood in the ruins of a synagogue in Capernaum, a spot on which Jesus Christ frequented while He lived on earth. I saw the ancient olive trees in the Garden of Gethsemane, and in fact, I walked in that garden. How can I ever forget the manger where Jesus was born and the shepherds' field, Jericho, believed to be the oldest city in the world "where the walls came tumbling down," the Caves of the Qumran where the Dead Sea Scrolls were discovered, and Mt. Nebo from which Moses stood and viewed the Promised Land? My eyes saw them!

The pleasure was mine to walk barefooted into the Dome of the Rock, and I saw the place where it is reputed that Abraham attempted to offer his son Isaac as a sacrifice. I saw and touched the Western Wall or the Wailing Wall as it is sometimes called. I visited the quaint little village of Bethany where Lazarus was buried, the Upper Room where Jesus partook of the Last Supper with His disciples, King David's tomb, and the old walls of Jerusalem. These places are to be seen, walked on and in, and experienced! I am indescribably grateful that those timeless places and things have not crumbled into the dust but are still there so that I, many centuries and miles removed, could be blessed.

As I walked around the rim of the Grand Canyon, I was mesmerized. Colors that defy senses and dazzle imagination were flashed across the Grand Canyon in rapid succession like an artist trying to capture those moments on canvas. It's very hard to describe the ultimate cataract, Niagara Falls. Literally tons of water have tumbled over those falls for hundreds of years, and its source has never been depleted.

The famous Butchart Gardens of Victoria in British Columbia, Canada, is a place where I imagine no one would mind too much to be held hostage there as long as you had the freedom to roam amid paradise. Acres and acres of gardens with fragrant flowers of every description perfuming the air are planted there. I just wandered with flowers, beautiful flowers! My eyesight of that lovely garden created images and placed them in a time capsule for me.

The changing of the guard at Buckingham Palace in London, England, is a marvel only the eyes can appreciate. There I saw dozens of trained military personnel with red stripes on their well-tailored uniforms marching to the beat of their drum corps and moving in unison. No one dare miss a beat or step out of line. In June 2012 her Royal Highness, Queen Elizabeth II, celebrated her Diamond Jubilee. That fine lady possesses such charm and poise that it's very hard to match. London and, indeed, the whole world seemed to have had a spontaneous burst of euphoria as she rode along the streets of London and as she waved from the palace balcony. I was privileged to have seen it all.

To behold Michelangelo's magnificent paintings on the ceiling of the Sistine Chapel at St. Peter's Cathedral in Rome and the statue of David, the Leaning Tower of Pisa, the Colosseum in Rome where gladiators fought to the death and where Christians were mauled and eaten by wild beasts, St. Peters Square, the Roman Forum, and beautiful romantic Venice where I sailed in a beautiful gondola meandering my way through a maze of endless canals.

I had the joy of being in the company of hundreds of folks from across the globe to see for myself the Oberammergau Passion Play in Germany, which to me was a small glimpse of heaven! O the wonder and awe of the snow-capped Alps and the postcard beauty of Geneva Lake in Switzerland! Those are places that poets love to write about! These are just a few of the wonderment of the natural world and the skills and architecture so lavishly bestowed to finite humankind from the hand of the Creator that I have enjoyed.

My ultimate must-see event will be when Jesus Christ comes in the clouds of heaven to take the likes of even me, to live with Him in heaven for all eternity! Just the ability to be able to see these letters on this keyboard as I write this book is simply a blessing! God, You have been good to me! And I cannot but praise You for the senses freely given to me, especially my eyesight!

Anyway, great-great-grandma's doctor suggested she be given the opportunity to see again by having her cataracts extracted from one eye at first, and if successful, later on, she could have the other eye done as well. That was music to her ears. After all the formalities of obtaining consent from family members and conducting preoperative procedures, she was ready.

After a few hours she returned to the floor with an eye shield affixed to the eye that had been operated on. Our bodies are fearfully and wonderfully made. Even though she had lost her sight, the part of her brain that controlled vision was about to pick up, to some degree, where it had left off.

As I thought about this patient, I remembered a story from the Bible that I heard as a child. It was about a miracle Jesus performed. One day He visited a town called Bethsaida in Israel. I had the pleasure of visiting this quaint little village in 1993. A blind man was brought to Jesus to be healed. Jesus held the blind man's hand and led him out of the town. Jesus then did something quite unconventional. He used alternative medicine. He put His saliva on the man's eyes, placed His hand over the man's eyes, removed His hands, and then asked the man if he could see anything. The man replied, "I see men as trees, walking!"

Jesus put His hands on the man's eyes a second time and made him look up. On the second attempt, the gentleman's sight was restored, and he saw everything clearly. This story is found in Mark 8:22–25. The story never said how the man lost his sight in the first place. I am speculating that he had some vision during his lifetime. He must have seen men and trees before to identify them the minute he could see. I wondered what picture my patient's mind made her *see* the first time she could see again!

As I stood there assisting the doctor in removing the eye shield and cleaning the patient's eye, she at first blinked to get accustomed to the glare. That was very good, and better things were just about to happen! That one moment in time was like a wedding on a cool autumn afternoon, a birthday celebration, and golden anniversary all wrapped up into one great present. She recognized her children instantly, and then she saw the doctor who had given her a brand new lease on life. She saw some of her grandchildren and great-grandchildren for the first time as well.

"I can see, I can see, I can see!" That was her story and dare anyone try to silence her. Granny had no plans to slow down, no sir! She had a lot of living to do and limited time in which to do it. Before we knew it, she was making plans to have the second eye fixed! The eye is referred to as the window of the soul, and it's a wonderful gift from God to be used wisely and cared for and guarded viciously.

What Happens Before the Last Breath Is Taken?

Life can be great if our basic needs are met, if we come to know and practice the word "sufficient," and if the fondest things that our minds conceive are materialized. What on earth does this idea of sufficient mean? I am no psychiatrist, but I am an independent thinker. I love to observe people, their facial expressions, the way they walk, dress, talk, and get to know who they really are when provoked or put under pressure and when called upon to do mandatory overtime! I realize that people are people no matter where we find them and that they get lonely and are often afraid, weak, vulnerable human beings; everybody needs someone, some time.

We need to know what we want out of life and when to put a stop to things when we have had sufficient abuse or sufficient stress that's just about to consume us. We need to know when we have sufficient money to do the things we have always dreamed of. We should know when we have put in sufficient years on the job and when it's time to retire. I also believe that patients know when they have had sufficient pain, tried and failed treatments, and when it's time to go. We need to know when to hang on and when to give up. These things make practical sense.

Everyone, especially adults, should state in writing what he or she wishes to be done in and out of the hospital should the time come that that person is unable to make decisions. We call such wishes advance directives. If those wishes are not made known in writing, chances are they won't be carried out, and people we have never heard of or seen before might have to make those decisions for us. Even though those wishes are, indeed, made in writing, they can still fall in the hands of unscrupulous, selfish people, so guard them well.

My ongoing observation of people takes me to what happens a few minutes, hours, or even days before a person dies. This is not a subject we like to discuss, but we all need to realize that this is really a fact of life, and sooner or later each of us during our lifetime is going to come face to face with this enemy, death. I know what it means to lose family members and friends, and it hurts—it hurts like crazy! Weeks and years sometimes heal those wounds, but at times, they heal with pain and big scars!

What goes through a person's thought prior to death? We always hear of that classic tunnel with lights, out of body experiences, and a host of near-death experiences that are hard to ignore. Some societies seem to embrace death, and during the days of the pharaohs, preparation for the afterlife was uppermost in their minds. I visited the Egyptian museum in Cairo, Egypt, and saw the treasures of King Tut. He went out in fine style into his "afterlife," but his body is still mummified and lying in a glass case for the world to see.

I have had so many patients who, over the years, have used different terms to indicate that they were dying. Some would say, "I am going," "I am traveling," "I am going home," "I am ready to go," or "I am dying."

One Friday I was working the afternoon shift back in my homeland. A patient with a chronic disease had been coming back more frequently over the last few weeks. He was admitted to the ward during the morning shift. As I made my rounds, I spotted him, and as usual I spoke with him and asked him how he was feeling. He was just tired, tired of coming back so often, tired of being sick, tired of not being able to take care of himself and his family as he would have liked. In spite of all that, he was able to work up a smile even for a brief spell.

It was soon suppertime, and I took him his tray. He told me he was not hungry and that I should just leave it by his bedside. I went to the end of the ward checking on all my patients. Somehow, I had this sinking feeling that all was not quite okay with him. He denied any pain or discomfort. I went back to him and asked if he needed anything.

"Are you sure I cannot do anything else for you, sir?" I asked

"Please give me a Bible," he requested.

I found a Bible quickly and gave it to him; he thanked me.

As the evening progressed, I checked on him again and offered him his medications. He requested that they be given a little later. Within half an hour or so I went back and this time he said to me, "Nurse, I am ready." I thought he was ready to eat or to have his medications, so I reheated his food and placed the tray in front of him and left because I thought he was able to feed himself.

I then sat down to do some charting at the nurses' station. I was in no way deeply concerned about this gentleman. I, however, got up from my desk for no apparent reason and checked on him one more time. The Bible was open to Psalm 23, and the man appeared to be asleep. I stood there for a while observing his breathing, only to realize that he wasn't breathing. I checked his pulse and blood pressure, and there was none as well. He was totally unresponsive!

I could not bring myself to accept the fact that the man had died in a matter of a few minutes after I had spoken to him. He told me he was ready, but ready for what? The man had given me a message, but I hadn't picked up the vibes. He was ready to go, and he went ever so quietly and peacefully. May his soul rest in peace.

One morning I got my report from the night staff that one of the patients who would be under my care was receiving a blood transfusion, which had started a few minutes ago. She was one of my favorite patients. Over the years she needed transfusions every once in a while because of her disease. People can react adversely to blood transfusions at any time during and after the blood is actually given, so they have to be monitored closely. As soon as I had finished getting the report from the night nurse, I went straight to the patient's room to see how she was doing.

She held my hand with a vicelike grip and told me not to leave her because she was going today. I told her that it seemed very unlikely she would be discharged on that day, seeing that she was still sick and needed two more units of blood. She still held onto my hand with all the strength she could muster and repeated that she was quite certain she was "going today"! Next door to this patient's room was a feeding pump whose alarm was loudly beeping, so I assured her that I would return to her as soon as I had checked on the patient next door. I physically had to prime my hand from this woman's grip.

Mission accomplished, I returned to see her. She seemed to be tolerating the transfusion quite well, so I attempted once again to leave her when she repeated the same statement, but this time she told me she was afraid and that I should stay with her. In the meantime it seemed as if she was trying to draw strength from me. It was still early into the shift, and I had not yet seen or assessed all my patents. With all my good intentions, I thought I could not stay with her any longer, but as before, I promised to come back as often as I could. This time she let go of my hand without any protest. When I reached the door, her attending doctor was entering the room to see her. As he approached her bed, he observed that something was amiss, so he called after me.

"Didn't I just hear my patient and you talking the minute I walked in and you promised her that you would come back to see her?"

"Yes," I replied.

"Well, she's dead!"

She was the only patient in that room so what he had heard was correct.

"What do you mean she is dead? That's impossible!" I replied.

"Well, come and see for yourself," he responded.

When I returned to the patient's bedside her hand was outstretched as if waiting to be held again. She had, indeed, expired.

It was very hard at first for me to reconcile the fact that my patient needed me, made several attempts to physically restrain me, gave me many clues that she was dying, and I never got it. What does it take for nurses and doctors to get it? In our zeal to have things done in a timely manner without compromising patient care, we sometimes have our priorities crossed. What could I have done differently? What lessons have I learned? A lot. I learned that it is not nice to die alone without even one person there to hold a hand or give a sip of water. I observed over the years that patients sometimes request a cool drink of water before they die. I learned that when patients tell me they are dying in any term or phrase, I take them seriously. I have learned to pull up a chair and sit beside my patients as much as time and circumstances allow. What do they see that the rest of us cannot see? This still remains a great mystery.

The "Something" That Disappeared

One evening I admitted a patient who had a lump in a part of her body and a diagnosis that every woman dreads. She was scheduled to have the affected area removed the following morning. This patient and her family were well known to me, so obtaining her history was quite easy. As the interview progressed, I thought that her behavior was a bit odd considering that she was just a few hours from having surgery and no telling what further treatment she would face following surgery.

Curiosity got the best of me, and owing to the fact that I knew her well enough, I took the liberty of asking her, "Are you alright?" She replied that she had never felt better.

"Are you aware that you are having surgery tomorrow and that the surgeon is coming up in a short time to have you sign a consent to have the operation done?"

"I am quite aware of it, my friend, but I must let you know that I am not afraid because my children and my church family have been praying, and I am sure that I do not have what the doctor says I have. The doctor told me that he felt *something* in my ___, they did an ultrasound and CT scan, and every test showed that big *thing* is there, but I am sure it has disappeared, because God has removed it. Nothing is impossible when you put your trust in God," she added.

Out of curiosity, I told her I would like to palpate the *thing* myself. She pointed to the area where the *thing* should have been. I began to gently feel the area, but I myself could not detect anything. I got on the phone and called her attending doctor and made him aware of my findings. Of course he was a bit skeptical because he had seen her in his office just a few hours before to make final preparations for the surgery that was pending.

"May I make a suggestion? Come over and see for yourself what I just told you. You can make your final decision then. As a matter of fact, her son is standing right here, and he is also requesting that you come,"

I said.

The doctor came, reexamined the patient, and couldn't detect *anything!* He ordered an ultrasound, but nothing was there! The patient was discharged and went home with her son that same evening! Before she left she hugged me tightly and told me something I will never forget.

"Trust God no matter what. He still does miracles!" I am a believer because I have seen miracles time and time again. Some folks will be quick to say that that was just a misdiagnosis. We don't have to be healthcare professionals to goof big time, but in this instance the evidence was too overwhelming to be ignored. What happened, I am not equipped to explain, but all I know is that that woman and her family had a story to tell to the world of their faith in the Great Physician who I call God.

I'm Gonna Walk Out a Here!

He was one tough little person. When he opened his mouth and began swearing, the devil would look like a saint. He put frightening thoughts in the hearts of the nursing staff when he was first transferred to us. What he thought had been his fate was translated into uncontrolled anger and rage. He had lost both legs over a period of time and was wheelchair bound. He couldn't be fitted with prosthesis because he was unable to balance himself, and even if he could, he probably would not have been in any mood to try. He was just an angry individual.

The first time I was assigned to this patient, I tried to put away my preconceived ideas about him and will myself to have a good day! With such a positive attitude, I was confident, ever so very confident, that nothing would go wrong. Well, I went to his room with a cheery smile and a warm "Good morning."

But the first response I got from this man was, "You come in here all spiffy with this smirk on your face, what the ___ is good about this morning, and what are you smiling about?"

"I got up this morning in my right mind, I had a good breakfast, got here safely, and I am here to take care of you. You know something? It's a beautiful spring morning, the birds are singing, and the flowers are beginning to bloom," I told him.

"Who the ___ cares? I can't see them or hear them. I can't walk to see no flowers blooming. Get the ___ out of here, you ___!" he said.

He used a few choice words that if certain militant members of one particular ethnic group were present, they would have physically dragged him from that bed and done him grievous bodily harm! All through that ranting and raving I never took him seriously because I knew he was just having displaced anger!

Breakfast came but what was presented on that plastic platter was not what his majesty desired, so he hurled that tray across the room. He was really out of control, and it was time to set some sort of limit to his foul behavior! I calmly walked up to his bedside and uttered not a single word. I just stood there. I was in no great hurry to leave; I had time. I waited some more. Do you remember the unstructured group discussion I told you about when I was a student nurse? Well, I decided to use that approach and see who would be the first to talk or act!

My patient took his first look at me. Prior to that moment he had never even acknowledged my presence as a person. I was just an employee paid to clean up after him, turn and position him, feed and medicate him. After all, his tax dollars helped to sustain the likes of me and the others who should be in awe of him!

"What did you say your name was again?" he asked in a subdued tone of voice.

"My name is Miss McCalla."

"What do they call you?" he asked

"They call me Miss McCalla." I gave him the information he needed. I was not prepared to have any small talk with him.

"Can I talk to you for a moment?" he asked. That was music to my ear, but I didn't want him to get any thrill from it.

"What do you want to talk about, sir?" I asked him.

With that invitation, he began his story, and I was all ears. He recounted his years as a young man living on a farm, full of life and vigor, riding horses and doing the things that he loved best. He later joined the military, did his tour of duty, and was honorably discharged. He got married, but lost his wife some years afterwards. He later became a free spirit doing things and going places he loved.

Life was good. He would drive long distances during the summer to visit friends and family in different states. One day he felt a pain in one of his feet. On closer examination, he observed that his toes were discolored and cold to touch. A visit to the doctors confirmed that he had very poor circulation in that limb and that he needed to have surgery to try to save it. Surgery was unsuccessful and before long that leg had to be amputated below the knee. That was a mental and physical blow to this macho man.

As the years progressed, his physical and mental health declined. That morning we had to fast-forward his story in the interest of time. He had just recently lost his second leg and that to him was double jeopardy. He was crushed. He began venting all his pent up anger and frustration at whomever happened to cross his path. I believe that most nurses would have gladly traded him off for 10 other patients. He was a nurse's greatest nightmare. Someone once remarked, "Can you imagine if that man was your landlord and you owed him one month's rent how he would *curse* you out?" I didn't want to stretch my imagination that far.

As I stood by that man's bedside that morning, a wave of pity swept over me, and I had to pause in my tracks and ask myself some soul-searching questions. If I were in that patient's position, in his bed at that point in time, what would my disposition be? Would I be tossing trays across the floor and making unreasonable demands of the staff, or would I have come to accept the things I could not change? I guess we will never quite know how we would act or react until we have a similar experience.

"Nurse, when I call you names, yell and scream at people, believe me, that is not like me to behave in such a manner. It's the pain, the anxiety, the self-pity, and the knowledge that I have to depend on people to do the things I once could do myself, independently. I do not mean to hurt anybody. Deep down, I am a real nice guy, you know." I could meet him halfway with his line of rationalization, but I could not accept it. Rude behavior should never be condoned. After he made that confession, I saw the most adorable smile on his face—a genuine smile.

I took the time to listen. That was all he needed at that time. I was non-judgmental. That man had some real issues that needed to be addressed. Granted, I got the blunt end of his anger, but as time went by, as a staff, we continued to chip away at that rough, tough exterior, and to everyone's amazement, there was a heart of gold, pure soft gold, hiding some place in that little chest of his.

Old habits die hard, so every once in a while he would revert to his old, mean behavior to get his way. If things were not going as fast as he wanted, he would yell, "I'm gonna walk out a here and never come back." In fits of anger and frustration, his mind gave his stumps legs and feet, if only for a brief moment.

This once dreaded patient, with patience, became our star patient. It was as if the nurses and aides could not wait to take turns caring for him even if he was not assigned to them on a particular day. He had a great sense of humor and a smile to go with it.

Regardless of how much nurses get attached to patients and no matter how attached they become to us, there comes a time when they get discharged from the hospital, transferred, or even die. It's not always easy to say goodbye to some of them. It was hard to say goodbye to this transformed human being. The morning he left we got his permission to take pictures of him and with him. My copies have gotten lost in the shuffle of life, but my memories of him still live in my heart. He never got a chance to walk out of our hearts.

I Remember You!

I have tried very hard over the years to sort of detach and distance myself from the hospital when I am not scheduled to be there, but it seems as though some patients do not allow me to do so. Every once in a while, some former patient or family member comes up to me and gives me a hug and kiss, thanking me for caring for them months or years ago. If I should confess, nine out of ten times, I haven't got a clue as to whom I am hugging. But why deny them the thrill of the reunion? Somewhere in time I must have done something good for them, and they never forgot. On the flip side, some do not forget the bad things they think they endured at the hands of the nurses and other medical personnel. Believe me, they rehearse those moments and occasions and are armed and ready for battle when the right moment presents itself.

I had not seen this one patient for many years, and as a matter of fact, not since he was discharged from the hospital. When I did see him some years later, I did not have any idea of who he was, but he had not forgotten me. I was standing in a crowded bank one day. A gentleman had finished his banking transaction and was just about to make his exit when he glanced in my direction. I could see that questioning look on his face as if to say, "Where have I seen this person before. I know you, but somehow I can't really put my finger on who you are." He walked to the door of the building then retraced his steps and came to where I was standing.

"You are nurse Milicent, aren't you? You took care of me four years ago," he said.

It was pretty obvious to him that I just could not remember him at all. His next question was, "How could you ever forget me?"

I was wondering what those folks in the bank were thinking because he was not particularly soft spoken. It was as if he had a story to tell and everyone had better listen!

He then craved an audience. "Listen folks, you see this lady standing here; I was in a hospital very depressed, and I refused to get out of bed because I was feeling so sorry for myself, and she *threatened* me. I refused to go to physiotherapy even though I could not even wipe my own butt, much less walk. One morning I was so down that I even thought of ending it all when she came to my bedside, pulled up a chair, and just sat by me. She asked me why I was refusing treatment that would eventually pave the way to independence. I never answered so she said that I was acting like a coward and a wimp! But she didn't stopped there. She said that as long as I was in her care, I was going to get myself out of that bed and start therapy because she cared about me. For once in a long time, I cried. She got the satisfaction of seeing me cry, and I cried like a baby that morning. She then had the nerve to tell me that by the time she came back to my room I would be out of bed and dressed because she was sending somebody to help me or I would never hear the end of it. At first I thought, who does she think she is? But I obeyed her because I didn't have a choice, and here I am today walking with a cane just for balancing."

He then turned to me and asked, "Nurse Milicent, do you remember me now?" I certainly did. I remembered much more than he volunteered to tell his audience. The pieces of that man's story began to take shape. There he was, a big six-footer lying in bed. He had to be turned and positioned, assisted with bathing and of course he was given bedpans. He became quite angry and depressed but not nasty. I think he vented his frustration on himself. One morning he rang for assistance, and I responded and gave him the needed bedpan. I assured him I would return to him as soon as he indicated. I did him the honors of cleaning him up under protest even though he himself could not do so at that point in time. I reassured him that what I was doing for him was part of the package called nursing so he should not take it too personally. He commented that he was very embarrassed to have me clean his butt to say the least.

I took the opportunity to play off of his embarrassment. "So you don't want me to clean your *butt*, eh! What can you do about it?"

He was unprepared for that question, so I filled in the blank for him. I pulled up a chair to his bedside, held his big hand, and just sat there. I like to find a few precious moments to sit with my patients amid the never-ending demands placed on us in any given shift.

"I will not fool myself to tell you that I know how you feel, and I honestly would not want to trade places with you. But the bottom line is that you are there in this bed. So what do you intend to do about it?" I asked him.

"What do you mean by that?" he asked

"Pardon me if I am wrong, but I am quite aware that you are refusing physiotherapy. Physiotherapy is the first step on the road to recovery coupled with a whole lot of willpower and determination to succeed. If you allow yourself to progress even to the stage of using a wheelchair or a walker, I would not have the need to wipe your butt. It's about time you got real and stopped feeing sorry for yourself. And there is one more thing; I think you are behaving like a child!"

Somewhere in my mind I asked myself if I had gotten a little carried away or if he would report me to the powers that be for insulting him. After all, I told him some pretty strong words! I also surprised myself for speaking to a patient like this. This had never happened to me before. Instead of retaliating, he looked at me like a cornered animal, and he began to sob like a baby. I just watched him let it all out. I then told him that real men are not afraid to cry.

I decided to push him a little further. "I am going to get your breakfast from the pantry myself. When you are done, you are going to get cleaned up and prepare to go to physiotherapy. Any questions?" I asked.

"No questions, boss!" he said.

Needless to say, my patient went down to physiotherapy for several days. What happened during the following weeks and months, I had no idea, but every once in a while I wondered what had become of him. The person who I saw in the bank that day was a healthy, independent human being. I accepted his hug, and I could see smiles on the customers' faces.

His parting words to me were, "No one ever spoke to me the way you did that day, but for once in my life I obeyed, and I am sure glad I did. God bless you, nurse."

I still remember that scene every once in a while, and it feels so wonderful!

Don't Worry, It's Only Heartburn!

My oldest brother was no father substitute, but he sort of self imposed that role long before I was born. You see, he was many years my senior. I grew up with great admiration and respect as well a bit of dread for him. He was a soldier and later a police officer, and as a child, I saw those folks as having the keys of prison and the law in the hollow of their hands. My dad was also a soldier and a police officer, but I viewed him differently. He was a milder version of my brother in behavior, or so it seemed to me then.

One New Year's Eve, he informed me that he was not feeling too good. Exactly what did that mean? He could not put his finger on what was ailing him, but he knew that he did not feel good. I then started to pull out some information from him to see if I could come up with some reason as to why he wasn't feeling good.

"Are you having any type of chest discomfort? Are you having shortness of breath? How is your blood sugar? Any dizziness, headache, blurred vision? Any tingling in your arms or legs? Can you move your tongue?"

After my litany of questions, he commented, "Now that you mentioned it, I am having a little tightness in my chest, but it is just heartburn. You see I was doing jury duty a few days ago, and I was sequestered for two days, and I never got the right food to eat, so my stomach is all messed up. The tightness in my chest is not so bad now. I just wanted to let you know," he said.

"I think you should call 911 right away!" I informed him.

"You nurses always make a big thing out of nothing. I am feeling much better now, so there is no need to worry," he assured me.

If he feels so much better, why did he call me in the first place? I thought to myself. As the evening progressed, I called to check on him. At one point and time he had vomited, and he was sweating profusely. I repeated the suggestion that he call 911 at once, and again he was very confident that he could handle the situation and that there was nothing to worry about. New Year's Eve was mine to enjoy at home, so I decided to stay up later than normal and watch television, but somehow I could not concentrate on what I was watching. So I called my brother again around 9:30 p.m.

"Be honest with me, how are you really feeling this minute?" I asked

"I don't feel too good at all," he replied.

"Get dressed, and in less than half an hour I will be at your door to pick you up and carry you to the hospital, even if I have to drag you out!" I told him.

It was one of those very cold, bleak nights with thick accumulation of ice on the windshield. I came out slipping and sliding and turned the defroster on high, hoping against hope that my faithful car would spring into action for us that night. I foresaw trouble and dire emergency while my brother saw just a little heartburn. I coasted down the hill to his residence on ice and snow; fortunately, the tires had enough traction to keep the car on the road. In a short time we were on our way to the hospital, picking up speed but being super careful. I did not want to reach the hospital by any other means of transportation but my own!

It's beneficial to have a good relationship with people, especially with your coworkers. That night I needed a lot of friends! I was given professional courtesy, and God only knew how much I needed it then. My brother was seen stat. The preliminaries were done, blood work, EKG, chest X-ray, and then he was hooked up to a heart monitor. As the night progressed, he began having chest pain, real chest pain. On a scale of one to ten, his was *a twelve*, the worst possible pain to experience. He had progressed from a simple self-diagnosed case of heartburn to a full-blown heart attack!

Come morning, New Year's Day, he was sent to the Intensive Care Unit where he was stabilized and where he remained for about three days. During that time he was scheduled to have a cardiac catheterization at another medical facility, so when the bed became available, he was transferred there by ambulance. On Monday of the following week the procedure was done, and he came through okay, but the results showed that he had multiple blockages in some major blood vessels and that he needed surgery to correct the problem.

His surgery was scheduled for Wednesday, but come Monday night he began having serious cardiac problems. Seeing that we knew his surgery was originally scheduled for Wednesday, his wife and I went fairly early to see him on Tuesday, only to observe a bunch of activity in his room. I looked at her, and we convinced ourselves that that ado was all about his roommate and not about my brother. Oh no! He was pretty much in the spotlight. We arrived just in time to see him being taken away to the operating room for emergency open-heart surgery. I felt numb. I was in a state of shock and disbelief.

I could understand the staff's inability to give us much information regarding what was transpiring and what took place overnight to warrant the emergent situation at hand, but it was hard being in the dark. We were directed to a waiting room where we sweated it out for close to five hours.

After a very long waiting period, the surgeon came to see us. In an unemotional and aloof stance, he matter-of-factly told us what surgery he had just performed on *the patient*. When he was asked about the possible outcome of my brother's surgery and recovery, he told us that he never had a crystal ball! He was just about to make his exit when I stopped him. I introduced my brother's wife and myself to him, expressed my gratitude and asked him to explain to us what necessitated the emergency surgery and exactly what the term he used actually meant.

I thought that he was either very tired, frustrated, stuck-up, or didn't care a hoot about who we were. He did what he had to do. His scrubs, gloves, and masks were taken off; the instruments were accounted for; the patient was sutured up; and the insurance company was contacted regarding his fee, so his task was finished! And then I thought, *How many times have I had similar days when, had it not been for the love of my job, I would have called my supervisor and told her I was coming in to clean out my locker and never cross the threshold of that lobby again?* I began to make allowance for him, but I soon discovered he was just behaving like a snob.

"Doctor, you spent several hours trying to save my brother's life, and I am grateful. For close to five hours we sat here expecting to hear a word of hope but none came. Now you come out here, use unfamiliar terms and expressions, and when my sister-in-law asked you what you thought his outcome will be, you told her you did not have a crystal ball! Surely you don't look like the typical fortuneteller or wizard to me! I think that that answer was very offensive and totally inappropriate. Now doctor, you are going to explain to us in simple terms what you did for the patient and your plan of care for him!" I stood my ground.

"You are a nurse, aren't you?" he asked.

"Why do you ask that question?"

"The plan of care sounded very familiar and professional," he said to me.

I never for one moment wished to identify who I was. I just wanted to be educated. He later got off his high horse and came to earth. Of course he was tired after standing all that time doing an unplanned surgery, and he had had a rough morning. He later smiled and the light broke. He drew a diagram illustrating to us exactly what he did. He told us that my brother's postoperative prognosis seemed good. He never had to look into any crystal ball to see that.

I was determined to leave him with something to think about.

"Doctor, you are right, I am a registered nurse. Today I stood helplessly watching my oldest brother on what seemed to be the brink of death. For close to a week, family members and friends from all over the globe have been calling me for updates on my brother's condition. The stress has been crippling. Every once in a while, we as healthcare professionals need to put ourselves in our patients' positions, and see how well we can handle it. It's tough to be on the other side of the operating room table or the other side of the scalpel!" He smiled again and thanked me, gave me his business card, and with a warm handshake wished us both good luck and a good evening.

Up until that point of my nursing profession, I had never gone into a postoperative recovery room or Cardiac Care Unit. There my hero was hooked up to everything imaginable. He was on a ventilator and looked the live picture of death. All those days of being strong for everyone else, giving updates and reassurances like I was passing out candies, stopped then and there. I took one look at my brother and just bawled. I did not make a loud disruptive scene because I didn't want to be tossed out by security, but I bawled and made no apologies for it. No one was going to muzzle me, no siree! I had earned the rights to bawl. If I had not bawled, I would be the next patient in that Cardiac Care Unit!

One of the nurses assigned to care for my brother began to educate us. She was spacing her words and speaking ever so slowly and very clearly.

"This is called a ventilator, and it is helping the patient breathe because he cannot breathe on his own just yet. This thing in his nose is helping to drain fluid from his stomach, and this thing in his bladder is draining his urine. He is getting a lot of fluids, so we have to know how much urine he is passing. Do you understand what I am saying to you, miss?"

Everything seemed to be going in slow motion; I tried to look as intelligent and interested as possible, but absolutely nothing was hitting the grey matter. Nothing she said made any sense to me. I was looking straight through her. How many years have I been taking care of patients on ventilators? How many times have I done procedures that seemed like sheer reflex action? But I was standing on the other side of the bed, not in the capacity of the charge nurse but just another person who needed some ray of hope. Isn't life simply amazing!

The nurse who gave us that brief education, then gave me the unit's phone number and told me to call her at any time and that she would be willing to provide me with any new information about my brother's condition. Before 10:00 o'clock that night, my brother was weaned from the ventilator and was breathing on his own, and his vital signs were stable. The next day most of the fancy gadgets were removed, and he was taken out of bed and given a clear liquid diet. The following day he was transferred to a step-down unit, and by the fourth day he was home! I believe in miracles because I have experienced so many and I believe in God!

It has been several years since the night that my brother's heartburn escalated into a full-blown heart attack that warranted cardiac bypass surgery! He has not had any recurrence of that problem. He had been uncompromising regarding his diet, exercise, and medications. He was a star patient in both hospitals. I learned a very important truth in all that transpired. Never take chest discomfort for granted. It can kill you! God gives skills to earthlings to be used to bless others. Utilize those skills when needed!

I Kept My Promise!

She was one of those patients who made her stay in the hospital pleasurable for everyone who was assigned to her care. She had fallen and sustained a fracture. Even though she was old and seemingly fragile, she came back from surgery with flying colors. After a few more days with us post operatively, she was transferred to another facility for short-term rehabilitation. That charming sprightly senior citizen made it back home in record time. According to her, that place was for old people, and she did not like to be associated with too many old folks!

One Friday evening I was preparing to receive a patient from the emergency room when I discovered that that patient was my friend who had fractured her hip not too long before. She was having back pain, and so she decided to apply a heating pad to the area for comfort, and unfortunately, she fell asleep with it. When she finally awoke, she had intense burning and increased pain in her back. She stated that the pain she was feeling was worse than when she had fractured her hip. The poor soul had sustained burns to her back with blisters so big they were hard to describe. She was in agony but still was able to smile through her pain and tears.

With all that loss of fluid in those blisters coupled with fever and sweats, her condition soon took a downward turn. She began having all sorts of complications. She was showing no signs of improvement, and later she had to be transferred to the ICU. When all options were exhausted and it was obvious that her life expectancy was near its end, the family, along with herself, decided that she did not want to be sustained by any mechanical means, so they signed what is called a DNR consent, that is, "Do Not Resuscitate."

Late one evening toward the end of my shift, she was transferred back to my floor. She had lost so much weight and was lethargic because of the medications she was taking for pain relief. I went to her bedside where her family members were keeping her company. As soon as she saw me, she lifted her arms for me to hug her. I did.

"Millie, I'm back, but not for long," she told me.

"I am going home in a short time from now, but make me a promise, whatever you do, don't leave before I come back in the morning," I requested of her.

She then raised her weak right hand and said, "I promise!" With that, she gave me a big smile and drifted off to sleep. I never really expected her to make it through the night because she was really very ill but who knows for sure what effect that promise she made to me had on her?

I could hardly wait for the next day to dawn. As soon as I clocked in, I went straight to her room half expecting to see her bed empty or a new patient lying there. One of her family members came to the door and told me that many times during the night they swore that she had stopped breathing. I went to her bed, and she smiled and said very softly, "See, I kept my promise!" She held my hand then gently let it go. By the time the nurse assigned to her that morning entered her room, she was gone. She died peacefully in just a few short moments after I saw her. One family member said to me, "My auntie loved you very much. Thanks for loving her back. She certainly kept her promise to you, didn't she?"

My Classic Collection Watch

He was a very astute businessman, and he made sure that no one had any problem identifying who he was. He knew what he was doing, and nobody could convince him otherwise. He was a very bright, intelligent man, but when it came to his health, he was too down in the dumps to even care about what was happening to him. Going for therapy to improve his condition was not too high on his agenda at that time of his life. He had better things to do in the office. In spite of what his big ego told him he was, he was just a very sick man. A very important organ in his body was failing, and without a transplant or the available treatment at hand, his condition would only get worse and worse until he would die, plain and simple.

I was assigned to this VIP, this very important patient. I informed him that he was scheduled for therapy in about an hour hence. He bluntly told me that he was not going. I decided to use the same approach I used on a patient I mentioned earlier but this time with more caution and tact. I was dealing with a strong-willed man who had no intention of changing his mind. Everything was in place to start therapy except his willingness to do so.

"The moment you walked through those doors, you were mine. I care about every one of my patients because that's the reason I became a nurse in the first place. I will not allow you to stay in that bed and vegetate when you can get help, so I will not stop until you get up and start your treatment. You will be picked up shortly, so I suggest you have your breakfast, get a shower, and then get dressed."

If looks could kill, I am sure I would be dead. He was too shocked to even defy me.

As nurses we have to know when to hang on and when to let go and how far to push our patients. No rude behavior on both sides should be tolerated. I use strong hands but a gentle touch, both figuratively and physically. I can most times predict my patient's response, so my approach is custom made to fit each individual person. Not one size fit all!

"Should I show you where to find the shower so you can have a long refreshing one before you go downstairs?"

I glanced at his table and saw some expensive looking cologne just sitting there.

"When you have finished having your shower, you can splash on some of those fragrances sitting over there. After all, nurses do have noses too, you know!"

That man must have wondered if I was nuts, a jerk, or just a comedian.

"Where can I find this shower, boss lady?" he asked.

"The pleasure is all mine to escort you there, sir," I said to him.

As I led the way I could hardly feel my feet touching the ground; I was floating on air because I realized that something great was going to happen. I knew that the mist that had hung over him for such a long time was going to dissipate.

That morning I volunteered to be his transporter. I took him downstairs myself to the unit where the therapy would be done lest he should change his mind and abscond! I managed to squeeze a smile out of him. It was more like a smirk. When I returned to my unit, the patient's wife called to see how her husband was doing.

"I just took him down to have his very first treatment," I told her.

There was silence on the other end of the telephone.

"What did you just say, nurse?" she asked.

I repeated the statement but this time more emphatically.

"What did you say your name was? I would like to know what you did to my husband. Do you really mean he went for his treatment?"

"Actually, it was quite consensual." I lied through my teeth!

"Consensual my foot! Oh no, you don't know the man I married. Nobody tells him what to do. He has been refusing treatment ever since he was diagnosed, so you can't fool me that he went on his own accord. I want to meet you in person and thank you. What time does your shift end?" she asked, so I informed her.

My self-made macho man returned to the floor after a few hours, washed out as he described his first experience. I told him that that was expected but better days were ahead and that he should even give himself a pat on the back and be gentle with himself. I remember quoting this famous saying, "The journey of a thousand miles begins with the first step." This time he smiled, exposing a set of beautiful teeth. I felt good for him and for myself. Shortly afterward he fell into a restful, deep sleep.

Toward the end of the shift, as promised, the patient's wife showed up accompanied by two of her daughters. They acted as if we were long lost cousins! They hugged me, a total stranger, and to my surprise, the patient's wife reached for my pocket and quickly placed something in it. I have always made it a habit not to accept personal gifts from my patients, especially money. It can have some great repercussions, so I steer far right from accepting things.

But she was so swift and it was so unexpected that I didn't have time to respond. I went to the bathroom to see what on earth I was carrying in my pocket. To my utter amazement, it was a jewelry box with a watch bearing the name of a famous television personality and actress! I tried to refuse the gift, but under much protest, I was assured that I could not be paid for what I did for the patient so I should just simply accept it as gratitude on their part. That watch has gone with me all over the place. It is a very attractive timepiece. Over the years I have received many compliments.

My patient continued his therapy voluntarily until he was transferred to a center closer to his office. It has been many years since that time but my watch reminds me of him and his family, and I often wonder what became of them. I realize that nursing is much more than going through the motion of giving medication and other activities related to patient care. It's going out on a limb for people who are so angry, frustrated, and out of control and who sometimes cannot see beyond their present predicament. It's putting our license on the line when we have a gut-feeling that our concerns are not self-serving but are genuinely geared toward helping another human being feel better about the situation no matter how bad they might seem. Those moments enhance a restful sleep for me after a long hard day. I feel blessed in so many ways!

My Speech Has Returned!

I am cognizant of the fact that not all patients will ever be grateful to us nurses no matter how hard we try to help them. I have had some who have a mindset to be disagreeable, mean, and downright nasty. Those seem to be in the minority, so I do not feel too bad when they show up like "blisters" after a hard day's work is done! On the flip side, there are those who help to make our task seem pleasurable even if it's only for a spell. The statements such as "God bless you nurse"; "I remember you; you took good care of my dad before he passed"; "It's so good to see you; you have not changed one bit at all over the years"; "You still work on this floor?" give me courage to go on.

The recurrent "I remember you" came only just recently. A patient suffered an illness that left him weak on one side of his body and speechless. Not the speechlessness that comes with shock or amazement like "I attended a play on Broadway. The performance was so spectacular and dazzling it left me *speechless*!" No that man became dumb! He lacked the use of the human voice. It was snatched away from him without warning because of his illness. I can't imagine how he might have felt. I, myself, do not talk too much, just enough, but when I want or need to express my feelings and thoughts, I must not be muzzled literally or by circumstances, no sir!

Some neurological conditions, for example a stroke or tumors, are like very silent killers. A stroke occurs when the blood supply to parts of the brain becomes impaired or cut off. Cells in those parts of the brain might begin to die. A stroke can affect how one thinks, moves, feels, or behaves. Sometimes the victim has difficulty swallowing, has poor vision, and loses bladder or bowel control and autonomy over other body parts. Well, this gentleman in question, he just loved to talk. He was endowed with the gift of speech, and he lost it!

When I saw him, my former patient, he began to give me all the good reasons why I should not have forgotten him, but I am only one person dealing with literally hundreds of persons each year, but I am expected to remember them all. I sometimes feel quite flattered and thrilled through and through! From the "Sound of Music" comes one of my favorite lines, "Nothing comes from nothing, nothing ever could, so somewhere in my youth or childhood, I must have done something good." Somewhere along the line, during my trek across the sometimes dangerous and difficult journey through my nursing career, I must have done something good!

The gentleman named the room number to which he had been admitted, the date, and the circumstance of his plight. From those glimpses I should, by his standard, have been able to fill in the blank spaces. As I listened to him recount his condition and hospital stay, I began to get an insight here, a clue there, and an "Oh yes!" there, until the last piece of information he gave connected the dot and made me remember clearly who he really was.

"One day I was trying so hard to tell you something. But my speech was advancing from nothing to slurred. That was progress as far as I was concerned. I was making sounds, and they made sense to me but not to anyone else." (We call that condition "expressive aphasia.")

He continued, "You sensed my frustration and handed me a notepad and pencil and told me to write. I became an instant scribe. You didn't have to write back, I did all the writing while you just stood there reading my thoughts."

You should have seen his face when he said, "You just stood there reading my thoughts!" He was as pleased as punch. Some weeks later he was transferred to a rehab center and over time he regained the full use of his limbs and tongue.

I guess he did everything to catch up on his once dormant tongue! I was happy to have seen him after all those years, but I had to run along because, if given a chance, we would be standing there in that very spot today still talking! The human voice in any language or dialect is sometimes taken for granted. We simply open our mouths and words just flow. We sometimes chat before we think, thus putting ourselves in hot water because the spoken words cannot be retrieved no matter how hard we try. But often silence can be golden. Some people are afraid of silence, but somehow I love the "Sound of Silence" as one famous singing group recorded many years ago. Very rarely do I feel lonely. I enjoy my aloneness!

We at times take our God-given gifts for granted. We can see, hear, talk, smell, walk, and feel—nothing to write home about. After all, are they not supposed to be there in the first place? Our senses are prepackaged and delivered at birth, and if any is missing, the recipient is labeled handicapped or retarded or slow. Yet so many of us get this wonderful gift-wrapped package to be treasured and used for a lifetime, and we take it for granted. Just when we begin to lose them we realize how blessed we really are. Let us take care of our eyes and our ears; let us exercise to keep those limbs moving and our hearts pumping to their fullest capacity; let us use our speech to cheer and uplift instead of spreading idle tales and gossip; and let's take time to smell the roses!

So You Are My Rival, Eh?

Over the years I have met so many beautiful people who I would have preferred to call friends and not patients. I have a special little touch for my oncology patients as you might have gathered by now. Ever since it was my good fortune to have been handpicked to open that center in Canada, I have fallen in love with so many survivors as well as those who fought valiantly but lost.

I had a patient in his mid-seventies who came in monthly for chemotherapy, and he would call in advance to see if I was working on his scheduled days. If I was not, then he would request to reschedule his treatment to coincide with my being there. Can you believe this? Talk about a man who had aged gracefully, a sort of Sean Connery, Omar Sharif, and Charlton Heston all wrapped up in one aging body! He was very intelligent and pleasant, and he got great pleasure out of giving me glimpses into his life and that of his family's. He was everybody's favorite granddad, uncle, and friend. He showed great progress shortly after he began therapy, and his cancer went into remission after a time. But cancer can be very subtle, and sometimes it returns full force to dampen the spirits of even the most optimistic. Well my friend was admitted one afternoon with a low white blood count, so he had to be put on protective isolation. His body was temporarily unable to defend itself against some types of infection, so we had to minimize his risk of exposure.

During the times we spent together, a good patient/nurse relationship developed. He told me of a time when he met a beautiful young lady and fell madly in love with her. The war broke out shortly thereafter, and he was sent away to join the armed forces. He and his sweetheart communicated by mail as often as possible, but because of his frequent transfers from place to place, soon all lines of communications ceased. She went on with her life and he with his. The war finally ended and not knowing of each others whereabouts, they met and married other people and had children and grandchildren as the years progressed. He told me that during those years he never forgot his first sweetheart.

The aging process and illnesses soon deprived each other of their spouses, and so each decided to move back to their roots. Coincidently, they both moved into the same building within a few weeks of each other. They were living on the same floor with just a few apartments separating each other. One morning as he was getting ready to put out his garbage, he saw the profile of a woman and he could not take his eyes off her.

As they both walked into the passageway, she had to make her way around him, but she was not concerned one bit about him. As they passed something in her gait brought back a fifty plus year old memory that could not be easily shaken off. After all, fifty years is a mighty long time. People change, people age and people forget. The odds of reencountering someone at the starting point of one's adult life is quite remote, he told himself, but his gut feeling kept egging him on that that person who had just passed had got to be his old sweetheart!

He told me that he had lost her once before, and he had no intention of repeating that heartbreak. He had a good life, a stable home for himself and his family, but his first love meant a lot to him. He did the unthinkable. He ran after her and pried the elevator door open. They were alone in that elevator that day and for both of them time stood still. He was not looking into the face of a seventy-plus matronly woman but the twenty year old who he had loved with a passion. He never missed a beat, but it took some time for her to recognize him.

Little did each realize that their respective families knew everything about their long lost loves and were secretly wishing and hoping that if they were both alive they would get together again. When you wish upon a star, we are told, a lot of good things happen. Their wishes did come true. They were determined to rekindle the flames that burned dim, because a spark was still there.

Just when these two senior citizens began to fuss over each other and to take care of the other, my friend was diagnosed with this dreaded disease. Their world was crumbling all around them. Heartbreak yet another time now engulfed them both. One afternoon while my patient was in protective isolation, a classy petite lady came inquiring about him. To my surprise she asked me where to find a nurse named Milicent. I told her that I was the person.

She smiled and said, "So you are my rival, eh? All I ever hear is this nurse who saves those extra blankets for me because she knows I am always cold even in the summertime, this nurse who always draws my blood and puts in my needles, this nurse who makes sure I get a good roommate. He never stops talking about you, so I had to see you!" She then knew that I was safe with him; there was no rivalry, no competition!

She told me her side of the story, which was so very similar to his. Like Tina Turner sings, "What's love got to do with it, Who needs a heart when a heart can be broken?"

She said to me that afternoon, and I can actually quote her, "I found him a second time, and I am about to lose him a second time around. I don't understand any of this. It makes absolutely no sense. Why is life so unfair?"

I was at a loss for words, but I said to her, "I heard my father use this quotation, and I want to share it with you. 'Life is not so much to be understood but to be lived to the fullest.' He is a very sick man, but try to savor the moments you spend together so far and those that are ahead."

The hug she gave me said it all. My friend was transferred to another facility a few days afterwards. I never saw him or her again, but I am sure glad I met those young at heart, October sweethearts in my lifetime.

Water Never Tasted Better; This Is Heaven!

Talk about a family who cared about one another. Time, distance, or money meant very little when they needed help and support. One family member became very ill, and at times I thought that his life weighed in a balance. When I met him he was restless and disorientated and posed quite a challenge to take care of. I would literally pray for strength, physically and emotionally, to deal with him during my shift, but I always came away with something positive because of what seemed like a miracle. Every day there was some noticeable improvement in his overall condition.

His illness left him with some cognitive as well as physical impairment. He had difficulty swallowing, and when a swallowing evaluation was done, it was advised that he should be given nothing by mouth because of the possibility of aspiration. Gradually his speech improved. Though slurred and slowed, he soon was able to express his wishes. At times it was hard to understand what he was saying, so when I understood what he was trying to communicate, he would laugh loudly as if he had just hit the jackpot! We at times played charades! "The beauty of any language is to be understood!" quoted my wise Papa.

One morning when his call light was activated, I rushed to his room because he had never used it before. His fingers were not strong enough for him to do so independently. When I reached his bedside, he was all smiles. Very slowly he told me, "I pushed this red button to let you know that I am very thirsty. I need a cool drink of water badly, nurse Milicent." He emphasized the red button so I realized that he was quite serious. Talk about a conflict of interest, this was a classic one! Here was a man who was as dry and thirsty as the Gobi Desert, but I had strict orders from his doctor not to give him anything by mouth because he might choke. What was I supposed to do?

All of my training told me to follow the doctors' orders, and most times I do. I would never encourage any nurse to do otherwise because her license could be in jeopardy. But I am a licensed practitioner, so I had to make a decision. This was what I said to my patient, "Your doctor does not feel it is safe for you to swallow anything at this time because you might choke on it."

Slowly and deliberately he said, "Please, don't be afraid to try. I am going to be okay; you will see."

I was stuck in a spot I would have rather preferred not to be in. I prayed a quick little prayer and asked God what I should do. Should I obey my patient's request or his doctor? I wet a gauze pad with ice-cold water, squeezed out the excess water and put it to his lips. He sucked on it like a baby sucking milk for the very first time.

He looked at me and said, "Water never tasted any better; this is heaven. God bless you, nurse Milicent" That statement left me misty. I repeated it a couple more times without any ill effect. The man was happy and so was I. I am not advocating neither am I encouraging any nurse to do what I did. I believe in prayer for myself and for those who are placed in my care. I know when to take risks, relying on God to help me help others. That simple act of swallowing just a trickle of cool refreshing water must have loosened his tongue as well because his speech improved noticeably each day.

Then came the biggest hurdle, getting him out of bed for the first time! He was a big guy both in height and weight. He had not stood in many weeks and had very little coordination in any limb, but he was determined to walk. I told him he should not expect to run a marathon that morning. Just standing for a brief moment would be good enough for me. He beamed with joy at the prospect of standing! A big, well-upholstered chair was provided for stability, and it took the team of physiotherapists and nurses to get him to the side of the bed so his feet could be planted on the floor. When we got him upright, he towered over most of us. He made one step, which he said was one "giant leap for mankind." We then helped him sit in the chair.

When I thought he had sat long enough and that he should go back to bed, he protested! With a wide grin on his face, he told us that he was not ready and that he was enjoying himself. He could not wait for the next days when he could practice walking again. I wish I could keep some patients longer than time allows because their presence gives strength. On the day this patient was transferred to a rehabilitation center, I was not at work, but he left a message to let me know that he would return. He promised that when he returned he would be walking, and he was holding me to the promises I made of cooking him oxtails and rice and peas. He was a vegetarian so he said he would settle for "veggie-oxtails."

On two occasions he actually returned to my unit walking with just a cane for balancing. I was not there. He was disappointed because he wanted to showoff his walking skills and independence! He and his family were relocating to another state. He said he had to make one last attempt to see me before he left. I was paged to come to the nurses' station, and as I came, I could not believe my eyes! My star patient was standing there upright and elegant with an enormous grin on his face as if to say, "I told you so!" I was so happy for him. He had to leave town in a short time amid the threat of a major snowstorm. I bid him Godspeed and continued progress. He never got his veggie-oxtails or rice and peas but who knows? Life is not over yet.

Cultural Diversity

During the many years I have been privileged to be a registered nurse, I have met patients from nearly every corner of the globe. I have cared for native Canadian Indians whose names sounded comical. When I first met Mary Roll-In-Mud, Peter Deer-Foot, Tom Ox-Blood, and John Kicking-Horse (not real names but very similar), I really thought those were just pet names. But those were their given names, and they did not find it funny to be laughed at.

But cultural diversity is nothing to laugh at. After all, I live in the city where the United Nations is headquartered. My country is represented there and so is yours. Cultural diversity may sometimes conflict with our own private and personal way of thinking, but as nurses, we shouldn't pass judgment on our patients' way of life! If people respected other people's boundaries, bigotry, racism, and malice would be unheard of.

Another observation I have made over the years, is the diversity of people's religious beliefs. Their God is real to them. Their varied vows and rituals are entrenched into their value system, and some would even kill to uphold those beliefs. I don't eat pork or shellfish. I worship on Saturdays, and I hold some other beliefs close to my heart. I know that I would not be too amused if my religious liberty was infringed upon. As much as lies in my power, if it's ethical and legal, I make sure my patients' wishes are respected and carried out.

I was surprised recently to learn that outhouses and latrines are still being used in places deemed affluent and modern. I was not too embarrassed when one morning a nurse who is far-removed from my cultural practices reported to me that during the night a patient in her care became quite confused and disorientated.

I had taken care of the patient in question the shift before, and she had appeared quite fine to me. When I asked the nurse why she concluded that the patient was disorientated and confused, this is what she said.

"In the middle of the night, the patient got out of bed, turned on the light, and looked under her bed as if she was searching for something. I asked her what she was looking for, and she told me she was looking for her chimney!"

I laughed so hard my side hurt. In my neck of the woods where the patient in question was born, the something that the patient was looking for was no *chimney* but her long-time friend, the lowly *chamber pot*! The *Oxford English Dictionary* defines it as a large bowl used in a bedroom for urination and defecation. That bowl is called by so many names, some of which I had better not mention here in writing, but the most popular ones are chimmy, chamber, and chamber pot. That poor soul was looking for something to relieve herself in. She wasn't confused and disorientated; she had to go to the bathroom!

Some folks who have arrived in lands of opportunity become so far removed from whence they came and are very embarrassed to talk about things such as these. I consider those folks as coming from nowhere! When we take a backward glance every once in a while from whence we have come and know who we really are, we will know for sure in which direction we are really heading. Even in a hospital setting, we still offer bedpans, urinals, and commodes to the patients who cannot make it to the bathroom. When we decide to "rough it" at campsites in the great outdoors, do we have marble toilets to flush after we have made our deposits? Life is real, so until we human beings acknowledge and embrace this truth, we are just phonies.

Cultural diversity takes so many forms that it requires a lot of patience and understanding to be tolerant. I have had patients from places on the other side of the globe who refuse to undress unless their husbands or other family members are with them. Certain parts of their bodies cannot be uncovered even to nurses. Who am I to judge, and who says that those practices are inferior or superior to ours? Acceptance, tolerance, and patience help to make the task of being a nurse or a patient more bearable. The famous writer Jean J. Rousseau penned these very beautiful words, "Patience is bitter but its fruit is sweet."

"You Gave Me Castor Oil to Drink!"

One day I heard a very "expensive" sound coming from the bottom of my car, so I took it to the auto mechanic to have it checked out. I then used the bus to return to my "crib." As soon as I attempted to sit, I heard a loud voice from the rear of the bus and a saw a hand waving frantically as if the person was trying to get someone's attention. Never in my wildest dream would I imagine that that loud ado was meant for me.

"Nurse, over here, over here!" said a woman sitting comfortably in the back seat of the crowded bus. I thought to myself that there could have been other nurses on board so why be overly concerned? Then she bellowed,

"Lady in the red sweater, I am talking to you. Don't you remember me? Come down here, sugar. I have a seat for you!" I was wearing a red sweater, so I was the victim! Was I being led to the slaughter?

By that time, others joined her in convincing me I was the nurse with whom she wished to reconnect.

I pushed my way to the rear of the bus even though my stop was just a few blocks away.

"Nurse, so good to see you again. I had surgery five years ago, and you admitted me. I came in one Sunday evening because I was scheduled to have surgery on Monday morning. You gave me a big cup of castor oil to drink. I didn't want to drink it, so you said, 'You either drink it or you are going no place tomorrow!' I ran to the bathroom all night; I never got a wink! The next day you came back with this big smile on your face and had the nerve to ask me if I had a good night! You might forget me, but I will never forget anybody who gave me castor oil to drink! A big cup too!" How big was that cup? I have no clue. To her it must have been a gallon and a half!

Her loud speech caught the ears of the other passengers. One woman looked at me with a big grin and pointed her index finger at me and said, "Shame, shame on you,"

It was so funny to realize that by following her doctor's order, she volunteered to expose her own patient's confidentiality on public transportation. It was like she was giving a free concert in Central Park! On the flipside, if I had done what she did, I would have to kiss my career goodbye. After inquiring about her health, she assured me that all was well and that although she didn't appreciate the drink, she was glad for my help!

The Young at Heart

One of my patients was a ninety-four-year-old great-great-grandma who was as mentally sharp as any twenty-year-old. On her nightstand were some books with very provocative looking covers! She was always reading and smiling to herself or laughing out loud. I got to know her quite well, so one day I said, "What kind of X-rated stuff are you reading over there today, grandma?"

In her Southern accent she replied, "Sugar, because there is snow on the roof that don't mean there ain't no fire in the furnace!" She was such a joy to take care of.

One day a doctor happened to pass by her bedside on his way to see her roommate . He said hello to both of us then pulled the curtain to attend to his patient. Granny was very hard of hearing, so she loudly said to me, "Sugar, who is that hunk?"

I told her who he was.

"I didn't hear what you said, speak louder." The doctor heard the query quite clearly.

"The Lord is my shepherd, I see what I want!" she bellowed.

The poor doctor could not stifle his laughter. He was behind the screen cracking up.

When he had finished attending to his patient by the window, granny began to engage this poor doctor in a deep, meaningful conversation.

"What is your name, honey?" she asked. He kindly answered her.

"If I was sixty years younger, I would sure give you a run for your money!" The doctor blushed.

"Never mind, sugar, just give me a hug," she requested.

Who in his right mind could deny romantic granny that favor?

I said to her "You must have broken quite a few hearts during your lifetime, eh!"

"You bet I have, honey," she replied. I never doubted her for one moment.

"Break their hearts before they break yours, yes siree!" That was her creed.

All This Too Shall Pass, Just Like Kidney Stones!

I had a coworker who possessed the weirdest sense of humor. He would say and do things that left people in stitches while he, himself would just stand there all straight-faced, wide eyed, and innocent. Laughter and wit help to defuse tension in the workplace that sometimes seems to engulf us. No one is immune to stresses, but our attitude toward those elements makes or breaks us. I choose to find the funny side of life and give and receive smiles when feasible and appropriate.

One Monday morning, the start of a brand new workweek, I saw this gent in the hallway.

"How was your weekend?" I inquired.

"Not good at all," he replied.

"How come?" I ventured to ask this comedian.

With this he began to pour out a whole Hoover Dam-sized mountain of gripes and complaints. I was sort of wanting to ward off the complaining, so I interjected with this question. "So how are you doing these days?"

"I am breathing," he lamely replied. "I know you are going to ask me about the kids."

"Yes, how are they and the missus?" I asked.

"Everyone is so-so, you know. The oldest is eight, the middle is five, and the baby, she is so cute, she is eleven months."

He took out pictures of them, and they were as cute as he had described. I returned his pictures, and he kept talking.

"You see that beautiful smile my baby has? She will be needing braces soon to correct her bite. She might even need a pair of glasses. Kids are so expensive these days. Do you realize how expensive it is to send kids to college? Thousand and thousands of dollars a year. I don't know where I am going to get that type of money. Gas prices keep on going up and up and up! Do you know how much money it takes to fill my tank, and it disappears so quickly! Just a few miles to the gallon. The last time it rained, my basement flooded, and there is rain in the forecast. I am sure my basement is going to be flooded again."

He branched off a bit to more dismal, melancholy topics. "I love my job, but they don't need us anymore. The field is too crowded. How am I going to pay my mortgage and care for my family?"

When I could get a word in edgewise, I tried to get him to think logically. "Your kids are still babies for crying out loud! Your baby girl does not have teeth enough to eat porridge much less bite! As far as college is concerned, they have a few more years down that road. Because your basement got flooded last time, it doesn't necessarily mean that it will be under water this time around! You are a bight intelligent man with a good career. You will always be in great demand."

He just stood there looking at me as if he was trying to hypnotize me. He quite agreed with me.

"All this too shall pass, just like kidney stones, painfully!" He had to get in the last word. With that, he smiled, "For a moment I got you there, didn't I, Millie?"

"You sure did!" I said.

In real life, some people are just ice-cold, wet blankets. They see dead flowers instead of living roses with indescribable hues. I have observed that some of these negative souls just love to rehearse their plight and crave an audience. "Misery loves company" for sure. I avoid them like the plague for before long, if I am not careful, I will be thinking and acting like them. My friend does not work with me anymore but I am sure that wherever he is employed, he will still be making people laugh, thus helping to pass the time of day in a less stressful manner.

Just for the Love of the Game

It takes just one tiny snowflake to start a mighty blizzard. That's exactly what happened one very cold February night. The weatherperson can be the most loved or hated person, depending on what type of predictions are made. "It's going to be a gorgeous day today. Please leave your umbrellas and coats at home and just enjoy the day." Everyone loves the weatherperson today. The next day the same beloved person comes on the television or radio and says, "Ladies and gentlemen, a band of high/low pressure system is moving across our region from Canada which promises to dump twelve inches of snow before it slowly moves out to sea!" Everyone is ready to pull out the shotgun, shovel, or machete and go after the innocent person!

When I looked out my window, I saw only the form of my car. I remembered where I had parked it, so I imagined that what I was looking at—twelve inches of the whitest, fluffiest snow imaginable—was my buried vehicle. All forms of public transportation were at a standstill. Of course, for the love of the game I had to go to work! Hospitals don't close down or experience a delayed opening when it snows! I decided to call a taxi company, but the person on the other end of the line, in a sweet tone of voice, questioned my sanity. I assured her that I was not crazy.

The previous year there had been a similar blizzard, and I walked more than two miles to work just for the love of the game, but I swore that it would never happen again because I promised myself to live for the cause of nursing and not to die for it! I was wearing a Canadian down-filled goose coat, which, as I continued walking, became hot as an oven. The road was slippery and icy, so when I made one step forward, I slid two steps backward. I felt as if I had run a marathon.

Anyway, I thought of my coworkers who were just about to finish twelve long hours and needed to be relieved—I hoped that they would, with the same consideration and courtesy, be nice enough to relieve me when my time came to return home. But I had no way of reaching work. Then the light bulb, like the ones that come on in cartoons, flashed in my mind. Why not call the cops to help provide transportation? At first it sounded quite funny, even to me, so I sort of laughed and dismissed the idea. Then I thought, *What other choice do I have?* I got the telephone directory and began looking up the number for the police station in my area. I found it and with trembling hands I began to dial the number.

"Hello, may I help you?" a voice at the other end asked.

"Yes, you certainly can," I ventured.

"What's the nature of your concern, miss?"

"Well, as you can see the weather is very bad outside, and I need a ride to work."

"What did you just say? You need a ride to work? Who are you, and where are you calling from, and where do you think you are going?" The questions came unchecked.

"My name is ... I work at ... and I am a nurse who desperately needs a ride to work. I live at ... As you might imagine, this is an essential service I perform, and I have to get to work and very soon too!"

"Woman, you can't be serious."

"You bet I am very serious. Are you the person in charge?"

"No, I am not in charge," she replied.

"Good, you are not in charge. Now kindly transfer me to your boss, thank you!"

I imagined that she was quite ticked-off because I could hear her in the background yelling to someone that some crazy nurse was on the phone!

The person in charge answered, and the same inquiry started all over again and the same answers were given.

"You see, nurse, it is not the usual thing for the police department to provide transportation for civilians." I thought to myself, *Unless they are being taken to the slammer!*

The voice on the other end continued. "The roads are very bad, and it's difficult for our cars to maneuver in this heavy snow at this time, but I will see what I can do." After a brief pause, he spoke again. "I tell you what; I am coming to pick you up myself because I really want to see who you are. It seems that you will not accept no for an answer anyway, so I have no choice!"

I gave him my name, address, and telephone number, but before he hung up, I said, "Do me a big favor, no flashing lights, no sirens, and no loudspeakers, please."

He laughed and said, "You got it!"

I made sure I placed my uniform in a transparent plastic bag so that if some nosy neighbor should see me being picked up by the cops they would not think I was being *picked up by the cops!*

After a little while a fine gentleman, young enough to be my son, came to my door with the biggest grin on his face. "So you are the person who left everyone wondering who on earth you were. I had to see you for myself."

He held my hand and made a trench with his feet to get me to the car where he placed me in the front seat.

I said to him, "Aren't you going to read me my rights before I get in?"

He just laughed. He must have burnt off a few miles of tires from my home to the hospital because the car skidded and got stuck many times. He seemed to be having big fun while my heart was in my mouth. He was trying so hard to keep that poor car on the road while the car was protesting and threatening to conk out on us. The car managed to make it to the hospital and the well-mannered young person helped me out of the car and wished me a lovely day. What a sweetheart!

I felt good to be at work at last. By the end of the shift the roads were cleared and traffic was moving along fairly well, so I had very little problem returning home. I ventured to tell my big sister, Yvette, who lives in warm, sunny Arizona of what I thought was my good fortune to have been given a ride to work. She became mighty mad!

"What did you just say? You were picked up by the cops this morning?"

"And taken to work, not to jail." I completed the sentence for her.

"How could you do such a stupid thing? What will the neighbors think? I swear, one day you are going to get yourself into some serious scrapes. The nerve of you to call the police. Don't you know how New York police officers are? Never do such a stupid thing again, you hear me?"

For a moment I thought we were three- and five-year-old kids again and that it was her good pleasure to tell me what to do! I remember picking a fight with her once when I was little. She gave me such a whipping, and since that time I have tried very hard to be on her good side! Occasionally we have had a few verbal wars but nothing that escalates into World War III! She means well and has always been my best friend.

"Are you quite finished?" I asked. "I know who I am, and I also knew where I went. I don't care what the neighbors think of me. I went to work safe and sound. I am back home in my own bed, and I thank God I will not be going back to work for the next four days. Do you hear me ... four long days? How does that sound? And by the way, what was the temperature in Arizona today?"

"In the mid seventies," she replied.

I hope that that need will never recur, but if I really have to get to work in any really bad weather, I know exactly who to call. I will certainly call New York's bravest and finest!

Saving it for a Special Occasion

I have had the pleasure of taking care of some of the world's best senior citizens. I just love old folks. Some of them are so shrewd and clever. I would have loved to sit at their feet and learn the practical things of life that made them the treasures they have become. I never met either of my grandmas, but if I had, I am sure I would have spoiled them. My eleventh commandment is "Thou shall never spoil thy children, but thou should spoil thy parents and grandparents."

I took care of a ninety-nine-year-old lady back in Canada. While she was in the hospital she was to celebrate her big 100th year birthday, so the staff and her family made a big thing of it. We fell all over each other getting her prepared to celebrate her very special day. A great-great-granddaughter had bought her a really beautiful dress for the occasion. When we attempted to dress her in that fancy new dress, I was quite taken aback when she said, "Oh no. I am not wearing that dress today. I am saving it for a special occasion!"

The lady was one whole century old, and she was saving the dress for a special occasion? How many tomorrows did she have? She was on borrowed time, but she did not seem to realize that. Her family and I tried to convince her that that day was, indeed, a very special occasion and that she should enjoy it to the fullest extent. She donned the dress as a courtesy to us but was not too excited about the whole affair.

How many times we as nurses as well as other professionals think about the day we will retire, maybe in our sixties, and then begin to live? We work hard and long to save for rainy days, and we see the future as being very secure. Then lo and behold we hear of our soon-to-be-retired or recently retired coworkers unexpectedly dying. The special events, the trips to exotic tropical islands bedecked with white sand beaches, and the beautiful clothes they had planned on buying slipped through their fingers like grains of sand.

Life is real; so is old age. We all need to invent some "rainy days," write ourselves a check or two, and just take off to some place we have always wanted to visit. Just go and don't give a second thought to it! The memories are worth the time and effort. Time, wealth, health, and memory are fleeting; we can lose them gradually or very swiftly! Remember, we can't take all the stuff that we amassed with us when it's time to check out.

At the end of each shift, I pause amid the privacy of my faithful little car and thank God for helping me make it safely out of the hospital. After many, many years of practicing nursing, I have not consciously or inadvertently killed or hurt anyone. We as nurses work in an environment where people's lives literally are in the hollow of our hands. The slightest error that we make can cause untold damage. So I celebrate the moments of my life and call those moments special. I deem occasions special when a patient tells me, "Nurse, the weather is very bad outside, but I am praying that you reach home safely"; "God bless you; you have been so kind to me"; or "I will never forget you. You took care of me twenty years ago." I celebrate in my own way a patient taking his first step after a stroke. I celebrate with my patients in remission from cancer. I rejoice with a patient who proves the doctor wrong by outliving his or her "death sentence" of having a limited time to survive their disease.

One of my patients was told she had six months to live. When the six months expired and she had not expired, she asked me why she was still alive. That question made me pause and ponder the audacity of anyone setting limits to people's lifespan. I suggested to her that she should forget the prediction and just keep on living and celebrating the moments of her life, for every moment is special. I learned that we should not deprive anyone of having a fighting chance or hope because that might be all those folks possess.

Why Was I Kept Alive?

I just love the great outdoors. As a child I lived on a farm and had the freedom to run from one end of that farm to the other without fear. In those days, the term sex predators never hit the airwaves, and I had absolutely no anxiety or dread of walking by myself on my little country road to and from school. I was told, however, not to accept rides from anybody I did not know or talk to strangers. Granted, I would have sometimes preferred the company of others but at times I had to travel alone. I never ran with the pack nor was I afraid to be different. Those moments set the stage for independence and self-reliance in later life. I rose with the sun and watched as it faded beyond the western skies each night. That was a very predictable state of being for me, so when anything happened to disturb that setting, it became quite noticeable.

My father took great pride in keeping a well manicured lawn and nicely trimmed hibiscus edges in and around our home when I was a kid. That was my world, and I could not wait to return there, even now as an adult, because I thought that that was a place in which angels would delight to be. One day my dad placed a plank with nails attached to it at the side of our house. That thick chunk of board was almost hidden from view by the thick hedges. My dad, I believe, thought that none of us would see the need to interfere with it so he just left it there and never gave it a second thought. But he was in for a great surprise.

We had a family dog named Rover. Rover and I were very tight. As a matter of fact, my first published book, *A Dog Called Rover*, was centered around him. If I got into trouble I would half expect him to bail me out. We were both afraid of lightening and thunder and firecrackers, so when those monsters were around, we would find each other and just hang out under some table or any other place we chose! One day Rover and I decided to go and sit beneath the plank by the side of the house for no apparent reason. To make matters worse, I began kicking it just for fun. Gravity has a mandate to do what it is supposed to do, so the plank fell on my left knee with the nail facing down. Thus, the nail drove deep into my patella. Rover's barking and my crying signaled that something was terribly wrong.

Our wailing and barking summoned my siblings' presence. My brother Noel extracted the nail from my knee with great difficulty. My mom later cleaned the wound as best she could, tried to stop the bleeding, and later applied some form of home remedy. I was given a bit of pampering by my siblings considering the trauma I had experienced. I felt really important!

By the following day I felt feverish and was not my same busybody self. I knew I was not in top shape, so I stayed in bed, which was not my style. My mother was concerned, but my dad, who knew me better than most people, sensed that something was very wrong the moment he came home after working at the wharf supervising the selection of bananas to be exported to the United Kingdom. Rover and I were among the first to greet him at the gate each evening when he returned home, so our absence spoke volumes.

His touch on my brow convinced him that all was not well. By then I was roasting with a fever and my neck was becoming stiff and my jaw was beginning to close up involuntarily. He knew that if treatment was delayed then I would certainly die because I was on the brink of having a full blown case of tetanus. In spite of the fact that he was hungry and sleep deprived, he got me dressed and headed to the doctor's office some four miles away. All my dad had in those days in terms of transportation was a bicycle that possessed maybe an invisible one-horse power engine and a rider who was in stiff competition with Samson, Hercules, and Atlas!

I remember being taken by ambulance from the doctor's office straight to the hospital because of the gravity of the situation. What transpired afterwards is still a mystery to me. All I remember is waking up to a pungent smell that I later heard was chloroform. Someone knocked me out cold because I had apparently put up a fight when the doctors tried to drain fluid from my knee. The knee had become swollen, warm, and painful. Strange as this might sound, the next time I smelled chloroform was in my high school science lab. The moment I smelled that sort of sweet smelling stuff, I knew I had encountered it before, but where? Then I remembered the knockout punch I had received many years before.

After the doctor finished the procedure, he gave me a tetanus shot. Within a few hours the fever subsided, the swelling was reduced, and before long I was my old self again. There is a flipside to this story. A boy my age stepped on an old rusty nail and had similar symptoms that I had. He, too, was taken to the same hospital where I was treated. The pharmacists might have overlooked the fact that their supply of tetanus vaccines and serum was depleted. By the time the medication finally arrived from another pharmacy to be administered to that very sick child, he passed away. In just a matter of a few hours, the medication that should have been used to possibly save that lad's life was administered to me, and I survived!

I sometimes ask myself, why me? Why was my life spared and not his? What kind of life would he have led? Every once in a while, I contemplate the real meaning of life. William Wordsworth once said, "The best portion of a good man's life, His little, nameless, unremembered acts of kindness and of love."

 I try to hang on to that concept and live every day with the realization that tomorrow is promised to no one and that I survived a potentially fatal disease and have helped literally hundreds of folks during my career. I have been blessed beyond measure. Every day is a cause for happiness.

The Butcher Who Was Allergic to Pigs!

I've had so many heartwarming experiences in my career—some are comical, some are bittersweet, and others are so painful I sometimes wish I could delete them. When I wish to have a good laugh, I do not have to go too far to get it. I just reminisce. I love to watch the old comedies on television: *I Love Lucy*, *The Carol Burnett Show*, *All in the Family*, *Sanford and Son*, *The Andy Griffith Show*, *Good Times*, and *Three's Company*, and *The Jeffersons.* These are among my favorites, but they are in stiff competition with some of the real live situations I have encountered in my nursing career. I am not sure if those patients would consider their experiences amusing, neither am I trying to poke fun at anybody, but as an onlooker, I see the funny side of them.

Shortly after I graduated and got my first job, I received a patient from the emergency room experiencing acute respiratory distress. The man was wheezing so badly that it was not necessary to put a stethoscope on his chest to hear it. Beads of perspiration dripped from his brow as if he had just run through a rainstorm. I tried to get an admission profile on him, but because of his respiratory status at that time, I decided to interview him later during the shift.

When he was fairly calm and comfortable, I asked him the usual questions like when the attack started, how long it has been happening, allergies he had, past medical history, and so on. He informed me that he was allergic to pigs.

"Pigs?" I asked.

He told me that he was allergic to dead pigs. My curiosity was further aroused, so I asked, "Did you say you were allergic to dead pigs?"

"Yes, I am a butcher, and anytime I kill a pig I have this attack."

My next question was, "Then seeing that you are aware that you are allergic to pigs, why do you kill them?"

"I only kill them when it is highly necessary," he informed me.

"So what was so necessary for you to have killed that pig today to warrant this major full-blown attack?"

"You see, nurse, I had a case in court today. My baby's mother is suing me for child support, and I am sure the judge would throw the book at me, so I had to become very sick for me not to be there. My father was a butcher, and when he died he left the business to me. I have no problem slaughtering all types of animals, but whenever I kill a pig or when it 'turns into pork or bacon,' and I get close to it, my chest just begins to tighten up!"

I found the whole thing so strange that I just tried to stifle a laugh, but it came out full blown. After all,

I am human!

He said, "Nurse, this is no joking matter; this is serious business. I would prefer to be in a hospital bed than in a jail cell anytime. I had no plans to kill a pig, and as a matter of fact, I did not have one available. When I was summoned to attend court as early as today, I had to find a pig and kill it fast so I could become sick!" Can you believe this?

He received intravenous fluid and oxygen along with medications, and he settled in quite nicely. Toward the end of the shift, his breathing had returned to normal, just like that! No wheezing, no cough, no shortness of breath. His lungs were as clear as a bell. The gentleman came to the nurses' station and requested that I take the needle out of his arm and that I call the doctor to "check him out."

"Are you for real?" I asked him.

"Nurse, let me put it this way so you can understand. It is now minutes to four in the evening. The courthouse should be closing very soon, so my case won't be called up for many weeks down to road. If the case does come up again, you will certainly see me again, so until such time, I am checking out of here!" I am not sure if he ever had his day in court. I immigrated to Canada shortly after that incidence.

Some illnesses are psychosomatic. This one was classic, I tell you. Some patients continuously complain of pain, and because they do it so often, some of us nurses tend to be judgmental or take them for granted. To those patients, their pains are real, their asthmatic attacks are real, their headaches and stomach pains are real. Who am I not to believe them? Until those patients are given alternatives, are reeducated to be less dependent on narcotics or other quick-fix medications, or are taught how to deal positively with what is eating at them, then they will always be occupying a hospital bed, and I will always have a job. Let's face it, we don't wish for folks to become ill, but we need to have patients! The mortgage has to be paid, the kids need their braces, and the doctors need to see us in their offices for our annual checkup. Life is not easy, I tell you! Having the ability to laugh at myself and not to take too seriously everything that comes my way gives me the energy and vim to finish a shift and go home.

Where Is My Daughter?

It was in my first year of training that I dreaded the very thought of being on my own and making split-second decisions after I graduated. At that time I was very glad I was not in the shoes of the charge nurse of the Pediatric Unit. I didn't think I could have handled what I saw at the start of the morning shift.

A little girl had become quite ill the previous day, and she was transferred to a hospital in the city by ambulance. Her father accompanied her, and after she was settled in for the night, he took the long trip back home, promising he would be back early the next day. I do not quite remember what ailed her in the first place, but suffice it to say that for some strange reason her condition took a drastic turn for the worse during the night. Just before the morning shift, the little girl succumbed to her illness.

The dad must have had just enough time to take a shower, fix his child her favorite breakfast, put together her teddy bear and sleepwear, and then get on the bus to the hospital many miles away. The contents in the thermos were still warm when he arrived. I was there when he burst into the room with a smile on his face eagerly awaiting a reunion with his child even though it had been a few hours since he last saw her.

Someone from the day before must have recognized him and alerted the charge nurse. The gentleman approached the desk and said to the nurse, "Nurse, I brought me baby girl here yesterday. I couldn't sleep as long as the night was. I fixed a little porridge just the way she likes it, so I beg you please, let me feed her myself. She must be very hungry now, and she won't eat with just anybody, you know."

After what seemed like forever even though it could be translated into minutes, the man was taken aside and was told the worst news he had ever heard in his entire life. He threw himself to the floor and wept uncontrollably.

In times like those, what can one say to a father, or to anybody for that matter, who has lost a child, a beloved child? When the shock began to wear off and he was more composed, he gave us an inside scoop into the four short years that he had with his baby girl. She was his baby, plain and simple. He was not a particularly young man, probably in his mid fifties, and she was an only child. She was his pride and joy—the apple of his eye. As far as he was concerned, she was a good girl, and he was very proud to brag about her for all of us to hear. He had bought all sorts of insurance policies for her, thus guaranteeing a secure future for her financially as well as educationally—her future was bright! Death disrupted all the lofty dreams and aspirations he had set for her, and he wanted to know why. A simple explanation would have sufficed.

I personally do not subscribe to the notion that our loved ones are in heaven looking down at us and smiling when they die. What's the motive behind those smiles? Heaven is supposed to be a place of joy, happiness, and total bliss. No tears or sorrows will exist in heaven, so it seems illogical for our loved ones to be up there watching us crying and grieving for them. Our dearly departed family members would not be happy in heaven if they saw the pain and suffering their death caused us. I am sure that it would have broken the heart of that little child to see her daddy falling on the ground and crying because of her!

I personally feel that when a loved one dies that friends and family need time to cry. I so often hear folks telling them, "Hang in there; don't cry." Don't cry my foot! People need to bawl and vent. There is going to be an empty bed, an empty chair, and a permanent absence and void that cannot be filled. Don't deprive me of the emotion to be angry, grieve, and be just plain sad! Those grieving family members need to realize that death stinks, but they should not go on grieving as those who have no hope. One day we will see again the folks we dearly loved. I long for the time I will see my dad again. I will have no problem finding him because his infectious laugh will draw me close to him! There should come a time to pick up the pieces and move forward.

I most often times approach a whole sad situation with silence. Just a visible presence or a shoulder to lean on is most times what those bereaved individuals really need at that time. Death hurts; it separates, disrupts, and makes life miserable for people.

It has been many years now since that incidence occurred. I sometimes think about that father. How did he cope? It must have been a joy to pick out the most beautiful crib for his baby at birth and the most painful task to choose a casket! Did he pick up the pieces of his life and move on, or did he just sit there and wallow in self-pity and depression? I hope he somehow found some type of closure as the years passed.

One time I saw a father who was the sole survivor of a family tragedy being interviewed on television. His wife and two daughters had been brutally murdered. He made a statement that has stuck with me. He said, "When someone loses a spouse, he or she becomes a widow or a widower. When a parent loses a child, what is he or she called, what does he or she become?" Thought provoking, indeed!

At that time in my training I was very glad I was not "in the heat of the battle" and called on to relay such a horrible message to that father. As the years have raced on to more than three decades of dealing with death and dying, the onus has not gotten much better, but it has gotten more tolerable. Instead of running away and using the avoidance mechanism, I have learned to be there as a buffer and a support system. It is said that one never knows the strength of a teabag until it is placed in hot water. We as nurses are placed in some precarious positions at times, and we never realize how strong we really are until we experience those trying times. We need to every once in a while pause for applause and give ourselves a gentle pat on the back. Bravo, a thousand times bravo!

I Believe in Angels!

I believe all human beings have guardian angels. I also believe that they sometimes appear in human form at the right time and in the right place. I have sometimes found myself in situations where I desperately needed help and somehow, out of the blue, someone just simply showed up to offer me aid. Those to me are sometimes my encounters with celestial beings.

My dad was a remarkably brave person and hardly a day passes that I do not take time to reminisce and find something positive to say or think about him. He made life worth living. On Veterans Day in 2003 he went to sleep and never woke up. May his soul rest in peace. In my growing up years, as a family we were not blessed with much of this world's goods, but we had a good life. We had the recipe for fun, and I hope we will be able to pass that recipe on to succeeding generations. We had a lot of love to spread around, and we had each other. Our concerns, shared joys, and sorrows have not diminished as a family since our earliest days up to this day.

Papa's dreams, aspirations, and ambitions were actualized as the years went by. He saw himself holding jobs that required college and university degrees, though he never set foot in any of those places of learning, but he got those positions and jobs and made a huge success of them because he *saw* himself there.

Not long after I enrolled in elementary school, my dad was given a position as overseer of a big estate in another part of my parish. We were transported into a fairytale like existence. We then lived in what was called a Great House situated on a hill overlooking parts of the property. We had so many rooms in that house it was simply out of this world to a child. My mom was provided with a full-time helper, and we had people waiting on us hand and foot. That was a thing of beauty! Man, we commanded respect and status which rivaled the prime minister and his whole Cabinet put together!

Papa never had any experience in running an estate, but he exercised a lot of faith in God coupled with copious amounts of commonsense in order to function. In a relatively short space of time, he turned around that large rundown estate into a thriving investment. Its owner was proud of papa's accomplishments.

The thievery and laziness was cut out. If it were possible, the previous workers would have stolen caffeine out of the coffee bean plants and enriched themselves! Papa changed the norm of that little tight community, which was an unwelcome change for some who were there long before his arrival and were determined to turn the tables on him. Papa had several acres of property cleaned, plowed, and planted with corn and peas, crops that were not too expensive to lose if a good yield was not obtained. It was sort of experimental. Much to his surprise, the newly planted crops showed great signs of becoming profitable. My father's maxim, which he used for himself and later drilled into us, was, "Give a little more than what is required."

Weekends were special times for my family. We made it special by spending quality time together—eating, talking, and planning for the week ahead. Papa was a wonderful storyteller. As a child I remember him telling us about King Arthur's Camelot and about the Knights of the Round Table. His favorite hero was Sir Lancelot. As a matter of fact, he named one of my brothers Lancelot! He would tell and retell that story with such heart pounding passion that we considered ourselves to belong to that round table where everyone was equal and important. Each of us had to bring *something* to the table, not food, but ideas and suggestions. Age, gender, or position in the family had nothing to do with it; each of us was given a voice. I loved those times because we were given a sense of belonging and importance.

But one Sunday evening it took only one mean, conniving human being to bring my fairytale existence to an abrupt end. My castle crumbled and fell. My Camelot was razed, but we rose from its ashes as better people with the will to survive and to grow. Dinner was to be served in a relatively short time, but Papa decided to ride out to see for himself how the fields of corn and peas were doing. In those days he had a big motorcycle that was as loud as it was speedy. Under protest from my mother and us, he promised he would be back before we took the first bite of food! When Papa said he would be back, we knew he would be back. His word was his surety to us and to the folks with whom he interacted.

Unfortunately, the moments dragged into hours as we waited for Papa's return. On his way to the site, he saw in a distance one of the estate's employees driving a tractor that was only allowed to be used if Papa permitted it. The man, supposing that Papa was coming after him to reprimand or even fire him, because my dad had the power to do both, maliciously waited until Papa was close enough, then he turned the tractor across the narrow deserted road so my dad rode headlong into a ton of steel. The man then dragged him into a ditch, which should have become his grave had it not been for my father's guardian angel watching over him.

Papa did not lose consciousness, but he lost enough blood to paint a house. He told us that when he looked to see where an intense pain was coming from in his left leg, all he saw was the sole of his shoe facing upward. His leg had been severed from the rest of his body except for a small piece of tendon that kept it in place. In spite of the loss of blood and the pain Papa was then experiencing, he managed to crawl up the steep embankment to the side of the road. He then wished and prayed that someone would happen to pass by and render him some form of assistance.

In the meantime we knew that something dreadful had happened. Even our dog, Rover, sensed it. He began howling and barking frantically like a wolf in great distress as we paced the long corridors of that great house. My mother had never had to face tragedy without Papa by her side. There she was as scared as a child with her children looking to her for some ray of light and hope, but she had none to offer us at that time. We all felt numb. Someone suggested we organize a search party for him, but where would we find him at twilight on such a large estate?

As time dragged on, so did everyone's imagination. Later we all went out to the front poach to see if he might be coming home. But there was no sign of Papa anywhere. There was a long driveway to the house, and as we stood on the porch, we saw a car speeding up the road with dust flying all around. The car made its way to the back of the house, and as we all ran to that part of the house, our hearts sank as we saw Papa sitting in the back seat of that car between two total strangers. It was quite obvious that something dreadful had occurred.

The strangers had been traveling on that lonely deserted road close to sunset when they saw my father lying by the side of the road. Papa was alert enough to give them directions to the house. They simply scooped him up and placed him in their car, blood and dirt and all. To this day, none of us can remember who those folks were, what they looked like, what car they were driving, and when they left! No one heard or saw the car leave! Those folks had to have been angels! We never even got a chance to thank them.

One of my brothers grabbed a mattress from the nearest bedroom and placed Papa on it as we tried to save whatever little blood he had left in his body. He was shivering like a leaf in the wind, and in spite of the blankets and sheets we piled on top of him his teeth chattered, but he never went into shock. Papa's lips were pale, and he was in severe pain, but he still managed to flash us one of his brightest smiles.

The news soon spread around the estate that my dad was badly injured, and before long a family friend arranged transportation for him to the nearest hospital some fifteen miles away. He was taken to a hospital in the city via the emergency room. An orthopedic surgeon on call took one look at my father's leg and matter-of-factly said to an intern, "We will take him to the operating room, and you will get a chance to cut it off!" I can imagine the intern musing to himself, *Yes, this is my lucky day. Boy, I finally get a chance to take off a leg. Wow!*

I can also see him through my imagination writing home to his folks, "Dear Mama and Auntie Sue, guess what, you remember I always wanted to be a surgeon? Well just last night I got a chance to cut off a man's leg. I could have done it with my eyes closed. As a matter of fact, I could have used one of your sharp kitchen knives to take it off because it was halfway off anyway. Be happy for me because after this experience there is no stopping me. Spread the news to the other family members. Love, your son, Joe."

But although the intern might have been excited, my dad was all alone, and that's a very scary place to find one's self. There he was, still shaking uncontrollably with the prospect of a prosthesis, a wheelchair, or crutches and no next of kin or a friend there for him to talk to. God has a way of working things out in rapid succession, which most times baffle the most learned and rational thinkers. On that fateful night there in that unfriendly city just about every bed was taken in that hospital, there were just a few stretchers lying unoccupied, but not for long.

Someone realized that after surgery there would not be any bed available for Papa, so she suggested that before his leg was amputated that he be transferred to another hospital! Just one simple thought, one simple suggestion set the stage for a night of miracles. Soon an ambulance was on its way to another city hospital with lights flashing and sirens blaring to let everyone know that someone special was on board and every minute was deemed important!

One of my favorite quotations from the Holy Bible is this: "And it shall come to pass that before they call I will answer and while they are yet speaking I will hear." Papa experienced that promise that night!

The chief of orthopedics was called in to see Papa, and he, along with his team, worked untiringly all night to try and save my dad's leg. All sorts of hardware was put in place enough to make a kennel for Rover. I sometimes wondered if he would, sometime in the future, be struck by a lightening bolt.

Finally Papa settled into a not so comfortable bed. Morning then dawned and X-rays of his leg were taken only to confirm that the bones and hardware were not properly aligned, so he was taken back to the operating room to experience a second round of hell on earth. The doctors were determined to save my dad's leg. They were there at such a time as that to care for my dad. God knew that we desperately needed him.

Papa was put on skeletal traction. The first time we were allowed to visit him the "nurse" in me caused me to ask some very bold questions. Papa was trying very hard to cover up the traction as best he could, but I could not help noticing that something strange was happening. What was that thing attached to his leg? So I pulled back the sheet, and a real nurse was called to give us some form of education. After all, what I thought I saw was a nail driven into my father's body a little above his heel with some sort of iron hanging from it. To me, that was a big cause for concern so someone had better give me some good explanation! My eyes were not playing dirty tricks on me at all. What I saw was real.

I still remember the explanation the nurse gave us, and when I did see a real skeletal traction for the first time during my training, I knew exactly what was being done for the patient. At that time in my young life I wanted to help Papa's bone to heal so that one leg would not become shorter than the other and that the bones would not move up and down and become disconnected from each other. In lay terms, as long as he could walk back into our lives I was okay. Those reasons were good enough for me. I was also told that my dad had to lie on his back for most of the time and that the weight attached to the "nail" or pin had to be kept in place at all times. Over time, my dad developed pressure ulcers. As a nurse, I hate pressure ulcers and try my very best to prevent my patients from acquiring them. Those pressure ulcers can most times be prevented with proper nursing care, but some occur no matter how hard we try.

As the days turned into weeks, Papa's fracture showed signs of improvement, but the pain he felt, especially at night, was always there. He shared a room with two other patients, a businessman and a minister of religion. He said that one night the pain became so unbearable that he wondered if the leg was worth saving after all. The minister and the businessman decided to do what any newfound friend would have done. The minister prayed a prayer that went straight to the throne room of heaven, and the businessman removed the weight and covered it up so that the nurses would not see it. Weren't the nurses supposed to have seen it? My dad said he slept that night for the first time since the accident. They repeated that little ritual for a few more nights just for Papa to get some much needed sleep and rest. The end product of that interrupted weight left the affected leg a bit shorter than the other. My dad would often laugh out loud when he limped at first, remarking that that was not an issue as far as he was concerned because he should not have had a leg in the first place! A simple insole was enough to fix the problem.

Papa came home to us with a cast on his leg and a pair of crutches. He got a hero's welcome from his family. It sometimes broke my heart to see him try to get inside his cast to scratch an itch that could not be reached. He devised a means of reaching that itch, though. He wrapped cotton around a piece of wire and slowly and carefully glided it inside that cast. When that mission was accomplished, he was so happy. That cast was heavy and hot! We made beautiful artwork on my dad's cast, which looked good enough to be exhibited in some fine art gallery. When the cast was finally removed, my dad's leg looked so small and flakey. We fussed over him, oiled his legs, and had big fun touching his hardware, which we could easily feel through his skin. A few scars were left on that leg. Papa would boast that he acquired those scars fighting for his life! He fell a few times but was determined to walk again independently, and within a relatively short time he did exactly that.

I still to this day wonder how my father's leg or even his very life was saved. He lost so much blood at the scene of the accident, and even when he was brought home, he was still bleeding profusely. It still sends chills down my spine each time I remember seeing the sole of that brown shoe facing upright and that leg dangling until someone placed it between two pieces of board and stabilized it. Why didn't he go into shock or develop some severe kind of infection, seeing that his bones were severed by old, rusty metals? I am powerless to fathom certain things, so I just move on, thankful that our guardian angels are always watching over us and that miracles do happen.

The man who tried to kill my father soon became a pitiful sight. He lost everything, including his health. On many occasions, Papa gave him food and money. He was homeless and reduced to rags. Papa forgave him and moved on. My father acted as if he had acquired amnesia. He simply forgot all the hurt that that man dished out to him. That forgiveness never lessened my father, but instead, it impacted him and his family in every facet of our lives. Papa lived to a ripe old age and saw the fruits of his labor and his children's children. I remember him saying, "Children of my children are twice my children." What a wise man! Where he got that thought, heaven knows. He must have read it someplace because all through the years I spent with him, he was always reading. As a kid I remember seeing him reading good books such as The Holy Bible, *The Power of Positive Thinking*, *How to Win Friends and Influence People*, *Think and Grow Rich*. He never amassed a fortune, but he was a very rich man!

I still believe that there are angels in this world who appear on the scenes at the right times and at the right places. I have no doubt that those folks who brought home my injured father many years ago were, indeed, angels. The nurse who suggested that my dad should be transferred, the doctors, nurses, the ambulance driver, and everyone who had a hand in his care, did what angels delight to do, caring for humans who need them most. I am, indeed, a believer!

I Have Learned to Hold My Fire

A foreign national who was on an exchange program was admitted with acute mental disorder after being in the bushes all day smoking marijuana and drinking overproof white rum. Talk about a volatile cocktail! Even for a seasoned user of both potentially dangerous mixes, it was hard to handle, and this was a first-time user. It almost blew her little brain. She was one wild party, I tell you! She looked, smelled, and acted as if she was possessed. She had to be put in restraints to save her from herself and safeguard the hospital's meager supply of furnishing and windowpanes. She busted out a few windowpanes and would have dived through if her head and shoulders were not so big!

Anyway, I was the night shift supervisor of both the male and female medical wards. In those days we never had male and female patients on the same ward. That would have been a prescription for trouble. A corridor separated both wards. In the wee hours of the morning, "a great while before day," I happened to be doing my rounds when I came face to face with this female patient. She had undone one of her arm restraints and was just about to undo the next! I quickly took a hold of her arm and tied it to the bed.

I turned on the light to check her arm and to make sure that she was okay. The little young miss must have had a pint of stale foul-smelling, sticky yuck in her mouth just waiting to be spewed out. Because when I got close enough she spat straight into my face! I held my fire, and I held my fire, and I held my fire! I counted ten times ten times ten! I used soap, water, and a harsh disinfectant to scrub my face. In those days HIV or AIDS had not made an appearance and hepatitis A, B, and C were not very prevalent, so the good old-fashioned soap and water did the trick. I gave no action to my thoughts, but my thoughts took a long time to calm down and behave and allow me to act sensibly. I exercised grace under fire. Every time that I pass through the doors of the hospital, I am in the "line of fire!"

Most times it's very difficult in any field of endeavor to turn the other cheek or to bite our tongues, especially if that cheek is swollen or our jaws broken. A quick fist or two in the jaw and a few missing teeth for the person who disrespected or assaulted us would appear to be the best thing to do at that time and then say, "You asked for it!" But I cannot do that and expect to sleep. Even if I was not seen carrying out my vengeance or if the patient was unable to articulate to anyone what I did, I would be tormented. My conscience has a big mouth, and most times it refuses to shut up and go to sleep. It keeps me on my toes and teaches me patience, which is a virtue and not a depravity. I can hear a resounding, "You have got to be crazy!" from many quarters, but taking things into our own hands most times is not worth it in the long run.

We as healthcare professionals need to allow the security personnel to handle dangerous or potentially dangerous situations. They are trained for those moments. We sometimes try to jump in to save the day but end up dead or wounded. I had a classmate in nursing school who was beaten to death by a patient. She was so badly disfigured that the funeral was a closed casket service. I will not be dying for the cause of nursing as I mentioned several times before. I have become accustomed to seeing blood all over the place, but I do not want to see mine gushing from my body. I promise myself solemnly that I will live for the cause of nursing and that I will walk out of any hospital on two legs and not be carried out in a body bag.

A story is told of a very pretty, die-for-a-cause queen who lived many years ago. Her husband, the king, never embraced her religious beliefs, but he was, nonetheless, madly in love with her even to the point of bending protocol to accommodate her. She was faced with a great problem that reached crisis proportion, and only as she placed herself in the line of fire, not for herself only but for an entire race of people, did she really realize the strength of her husband's undying love for her. She was a queen in her own right and wielded some measure of influence, but someone close to her husband was hell-bent on destroying her by any means possible.

Her commoner cousin who had raised her as his own child gave her something to think about. Sometimes all we humans need to change our lives and our course of action is some ideas to stop and think about. So this queen named Esther never became cocky or ungrateful for the kindness Mordecai showed to her during her growing up years. She listened to her dear cousin as he told her that her becoming queen was not by accident or chance. He knew that somehow she would be able to find a way out of the plot to exterminate her race. He said to her, "Who knows why you have come to the kingdom for such a time as this?"

She championed the cause of her people, and the perpetrator was exposed and eventually hanged on the same gallows that he had engineered for someone else. His plans backfired.

Who knows why we, the unsung heroes and heroines, came into nursing at such a time as this. We could have gone into other fields and became rich overnight, rubbing shoulders with the very rich and famous, but we chose to be nurses! We give hope, inspire hope, hold hands, wipe feverish brows, receive new lives into this world, and say goodbye to others as they die.

Nursing is one big adventure. Most of us didn't have a clue as to what we were getting ourselves into, but when we did, we hung on for dear life because we decided to put our hand to the plow and we refuse to let go. We should every once in a while ask ourselves some soul-searching questions. "Did I make a difference in someone's life during the course of my shift? What about last month or last year? Am I a hindrance or an asset to my profession? Am I helping suffering humanity or am I helping humanity suffer?" Good nurses and good doctors are fast becoming endangered species. We have to protect caring healthcare professionals the same way we protect wildlife, thus saving humans on our planet.

Chapter Nineteen

My Great Comrades-In-Arms

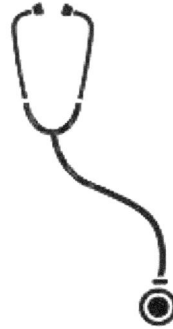

I am going to attempt a mammoth task. I am going to attempt to salute my comrades-in-arms, my fellow nurses. I mentioned some time ago that all nurses speak the same language regardless of our native tongues. Nursing, over the decades, has broadened its scope of practice and has launched into many new and exciting fields and specialties. From the halls of John Hopkins University, Sloan Kettering Hospital, Andrews Memorial Hospital, Westchester Medical Center, or Mt. Vernon Hospital in Mt. Vernon, New York, to the less talked about or even obscure clinics, sanitariums, and hospitals scattered in almost every corner of the globe, you can find nurses playing a vital role in the preservation of lives. We are blessed with the gift of healing not always by supernatural means but by skill, knowledge, commonsense, and the tenacity to fight and hold on to our calling.

What do we do in our chosen specialties? Why do we do what we do? I have never interviewed my fellow colleagues, but I think that if I should speak for them probably the majority of them would sanction what I have to say. This chapter is dedicated to nurses in the wide variety of areas that we work in. I have done my best to portray each specialty accurately.

Oncology Nurses

I will start with my specialty. A popular saying in my country goes something like this, "Parson christens his child first," so I am going to brag about mine first. Medical/surgical/oncology nursing calls for a double dose of compassion, stamina, and the ability to hold on and let go when faced with death. I once attended a cancer symposium in Canada many years ago. The keynote speaker was supposed to speak on topic of "What is cancer?" But I remember him saying that morning, "Ladies and gentlemen, I could finish my speech using a one-liner, 'I don't really know what it is!' We know the definition but what really is this monster?"

Can anyone tame it? Can anyone predict who will be the next victim? It is just a fast multiplication of malignant cells that destroys healthy tissues. Sometimes it lies dormant like a lull in a storm only to rear its ugly head sometime down the road.

Oncology nurses are in the frontline in the war against cancer by administering treatment and teaching preventative measures, and when all else fails, we hang in there with our patients and their loved ones. Chemotherapy is one of the many methods we use in trying to destroy this disease. We have to exercise the utmost precaution when administering this treatment both to ourselves and our patients. In our zeal to help our cancer patients, we are also at risk of exposure to the toxic chemicals used if we are not vigilant. Like most other forms of treatment that nurses and doctors give, the benefits sometimes outweigh the risks, and believe me, chemotherapy, radiotherapy, immunotherapy, bone marrow transplants, and other treatment options are risky business, and so is cancer!

I once had a patient who was receiving chemotherapy. She was everybody's favorite patient on the unit. When she smiled, she warmed up the whole place. She was on her way to the bathroom one afternoon when she slipped a little, and by sheer reflex, she grabbed onto the pole on which her chemotherapy was hung. In doing so, she dislodged the tubing from the bottle. Fortunately the treatment was just about finished, but there was enough fluid remaining to cause a noticeable spill on the floor.

The staff had to clean up that spill using protective gear. Her comment to me afterwards was so touching and thought-provoking that for the first time in my oncology experience I really stopped in my tracks and pondered what she said. "I observe how you all were wearing protective clothing, goggles, and gloves to clean up just a relatively small amount of chemotherapy spilled on the floor. What about me? I am receiving all those chemical in my body? I cannot run away from it; I cannot use any type of cleanser to get rid of it. Where do I go from here?"

It's the sad truth, isn't it? But sometimes the only recourse or treatment option is chemotherapy. Like all other forms of medications, the side effects as spelled out by the pharmaceutical companies can be frightening, but patients have to be made aware of what the risks and benefits are. If life is what we desire, then we sometimes have to choose medications or death. Alternative medicine is on the rise, and I have been cognizant of the fact that "belief kills and belief cures" depending on the individual.

Emergency Room Nurses

There are certain specialties in nursing that I would not be caught dead doing, and one of many is working in the ER. My comrades-in-arms are always in the line of fire! They do not know what to expect from one minute to the next. Some folks use the ER as a means of getting some form of treatment because of many and varied reasons, while for others it a matter of life and death. When we hear the familiar sounds of the police and ambulance and sometimes fire truck sirens heading for the ER parking lot, I imagine that those nurses get an adrenaline rush and gear themselves to expect just about any type of casualty. They are resourceful, strong, courageous, and skillful enough to handle just about everything! Bravo! They act and think on their feet because many a time death stares them in the face, and the split-second decisions they make, make all the difference.

They seem to "sniff" out veins or use radar to get intravenous access into patients who need fluids badly or who need to give blood to determine the type of treatment they need. Some folks do not have the wherewithal to start any type of intravenous therapy, but ER nurses seem to know where to find them! Talk about blood and body fluids; they have to face these every day. Lice and bedbug infestations are not unusual for ER nurses to handle.

Very rarely are patients turned away from any ER. They have to be seen, and if some of them are not seen fast enough, they can cause quite a scene! Most of those nurses are no-nonsense personalities though! They are not necessarily cold or callous, but they have to be on top of things before things get out of hand.

Who knows when the next train or airplane crash or the next terrorist attack will occur? When will a mentally deranged person or some bad individual decide to walk in and blow off a few heads? Whatever happens, ER nurses will be there, and trust me, they will deliver! And after they have patients stabilized, I am more than happy to take their patients off of their hands.

Operating Room and Recovery Room Nurses

The operating room, or the operating theater as our British counterparts call it, can be as unpredictable as the ER itself. Most often they have planned surgeries, but many a time emergency surgeries they never bargained for in terms of scope and duration arise. Patients come in through the ER or from the regular floors and need immediate surgical intervention. Thus those OR nurses have to be in a state of readiness. They prepare patients, stand by the surgeons, actively participate in all types of surgical procedures, support the family members, and stand ceaseless hours without bathroom privileges. No wonder they, as well as nurses in all specialties, sometimes come down with urinary tract infections, constipation, or varicose veins!

Many noteworthy procedures are done daily in operating rooms across the globe, and no matter how skillful those doctors are, nurses are there to assist them every step of the way. Open heart surgeries, separation of conjoined twins and other delicate neurological surgeries, organ transplants, you name it, OR nurses are there. Some of them have been there so long and are so knowledgeable and artful that they could teach some doctors a thing or two! Honest-to-goodness doctors would not hesitate to compliment them.

Just across from the operating room are another group of fine nurses who pick up where the OR nurses stop. They are the recovery room nurses. They are there to make sure that patients who recently left the OR are closely monitored until they are stabilized and can be transferred to the ICU/PCU, the regular floors, or home. They have an awesome responsibility because some patients take a turn for the worst shortly after some surgeries. Those nurses see to the comfort of those patients by administering analgesics as needed, protecting them, and making sure all is well. I don't particularly like those areas of nursing but nonetheless, I follow through where operating room and recovery room nurses leave off. You see how interdependent we all are of one another?

Intensive Care/Telemetry Unit Nurses

Nurses are trained to function efficiently in all areas of specialty. Intensive care and telemetry nurses are some of the finest nurses in the business. When patients whose condition deteriorates to the point I can no longer care for them on the regular medical/surgical floor, I am relieved to transfer such a patient to the ICU where nurses who are skilled and knowledgeable about such cases can closely monitor the patient. They attach all sorts of monitors and medical gadgets to patients as those very ill folks and their family members pray and hope for a speedy recovery.

Some patients leave the recovery room and go straight to the ICU. Nurses on the Telemetry Unit are at the forefront of monitoring patients with cardiac problems. Patients are hooked up to cardiac monitors, and doctors are immediately notified of any changes in a patient's status. Often those nurses do not have as many patients as the nurses on other floors because as the name of their specialty implies, they deliver intensive care to acutely ill patients, and it would be physically impossible to deliver that type of care with many patients at any given time.

The beds in ICU are very costly and very precious, so when those nurses stabilize their critically ill patients, I take them off their hands with pleasure as I do for my OR, recovery room, and ER counterparts. You see how important we all are? We need one another for the good of our fellow human beings.

Labor and Delivery Nurses

Midwifery has been around since Adam helped to deliver his son Cain! I guess we would have given him a different title, mid-husband? I'm guessing that Eve must have needed some sort of assistance during her pregnancy up until her labor and delivery period. In my mind's eye, I see Adam sweating while he gives Eve instructions to push and bear down until his firstborn appeared on this earth. I imagine that when Adam severed the umbilical cord, maybe using a flint stone, he held up his son who was wailing and making his presence heard in this vast universe. He had a perfect Apgar score of ten!

I also imagine Adam holding up his son and saying to Eve, "Look at that chin and deep set eyes; he is the splitting image of his old man. Isn't he just handsome? I can't wait for him to grow up because I have great plans for his life. That's my boy! I ought to call him AJ, Adam Junior. No, on second thought I will name him Cain."

Cain was the first recorded human birth on this earth, so he holds a record that cannot be broken. On this planet a baby is born every few minutes, and there is usually someone there directing the show whether it be in a professionally structured environment like a clinic or a hospital or some place in the bush. The focus is usually on the welfare of both baby and mother. This is where my comrades-in-arms play a pivotal role. Those trained midwives along with other nurses who work in the Labor and Delivery Units give their all to ensure the safe passage from labor to delivery and beyond.

Although we have all sorts of fancy gadgets to tell us of the progress or lack of progress that the unborn child is making and even its gender, I still love the waiting period right down to the last minute. I love delayed gratification! Don't tell me the sex of the baby. I still like to hear, "It's a boy!" or "It's a girl!"

I think that men have a sense of pride when they have a son especially if the first one is indeed a boy, but for others their daughters will always be "Daddy's little girl." They visualize the day when they will walk down the aisle to place their daughter's hands in the hands of the man of her choosing. Some even see shotguns in the horizon for any Mr. Man who dares to think of abusing his daughter in one form or another.

I assume that couples who plan to have children and after many years of not being able to produce any but who finally get the desire of their hearts must be the happiest folks on this side of heaven! The nurses in labor and delivery who witness those crowning moments must experience pleasure beyond belief for those happy couples. On the flipside there are moments when happiness fades into grief when a baby is delivered and some form of abnormality or defect is detected or a baby expires soon after birth or is even delivered dead. It must be very emotionally traumatic to leave a hospital with a death certificate instead of a birth certificate!

Those, I believe are the most dreadful times in the career of those nurses.

Or course, nurses come to the rescue of first-time moms who have no clue how to hold, feed, change, or bathe a newborn infant. Newborns sometimes seem so pink and fragile, but they are not as frail as we often believe them to be. Soon those brand new moms become pros and can't wait to check out and enter the real world.

A few years ago fathers had no place in the delivery room. Nowadays everyone and everything is permissible. Video cameras and cell phone cameras are there as if a major motion picture is being filmed. I guess the family members need to have memories to last a lifetime, but I am not sure how comfortable I would be as a nurse or as a mom in labor. But that's a different story.

Then there are other women who just love having babies. I once met a patient who had a dozen children. Although she was terminally ill, she managed to maintain her sense of humor and her good looks. Curiosity got the best of me, so I asked her why she had so many kids! She smiled and remarked, "When I had my first child, he was so handsome, pleasant, and cute, so I could not wait to have the next, then the next, then the next. Soon I had twelve before I realized what was happening. After all, I was pregnant for only nine months, you know. I had three months free each time!" I happened to see all twelve adult children together at one time and in one place, and I, at that time knew what she was talking about, such a beautiful dozen!

New baby care instructions, verbally as well as written, are given to parents, and don't forget the baby's car seat because that baby is not leaving the hospital without it! That's a state law, and no one is exempt! If you don't find one by any means possible, that baby will be growing up right there in that hospital! If you live across the street from the hospital, chances are, we might allow you to walk home with your brand new baby in your arms. Good luck, mom and dad!

Pediatric Nurses

I love kids of all ages. I never tried to have any, but I have dozens of them! Paradoxical, isn't it? My friends' children along with my nieces and nephews are all my children. Now that I am no longer a young spring chicken, even the interns, residents, nurses, and other coworkers sometimes affectionately call me "Mom," and I feel humbly proud to be called by that term of endearment. As I said before, I love children, but it would have been a challenge for me to care for sick children on a daily basis. I believe children are not supposed to be sick. They don't deserve to be sick! I cannot change the world or the things that often cause pain and suffering, but in the meantime, I steer far right from those things that distress me. I tell myself I don't have to choose pediatric nursing as a specialty because there will always be nurses who would choose nothing else. I really admire them for doing so.

How does one answer a child's concerns regarding illnesses, death, suffering? How do nurses cope with a sick child who cries constantly for his mom, especially at night when separation anxiety sets in? How does a nurse care for a preemie whose whole body is hardly bigger than her fist? Those and many other questions have played in my mind all through the years I have been a nurse, and I am not equipped to answer those burning questions. I know that there will always be my comrades-in-arms who will rally to the task of caring for those precious children. Heaven bless them!

I greatly admire pediatric nurses who are there every day caring for sick children from all walks of life with many and varied illnesses. Some of them are real mother substitutes. Within pediatrics are specialties just as with adults. It is gratifying to see miracles performed before our very eyes. Sometimes babies are kept alive, and not so much by medical or surgical interventions but by the touch of human hands and the human spirit. Pediatric nurses are there to stroke, touch, medicate, rock, sing, hug, and go far beyond what their paychecks require them to do in order to care for those little ones and not so little ones.

Those nurses are equipped with patience, skill, and the tenacity to hang on in spite of the moments when it seems near impossible to hold on. They have strong hands but a gently touch, indeed, and a heart big enough to encircle those young ones with love indescribable. I believe that most parents hold them in high esteem. After all, who else can they turn to when their children are ill? Some children practically grow up in hospitals because of recurrent illnesses, and some of those same nurses watch them grow up as well. It's like coming home to family on each admission. Nurses in every floor and in every specialty within pediatrics hang in there—we need you and no one else can fill your slots.

Geriatric Nurses

People are living longer and healthier these days, and so our senior citizens will be with us for a long, long time. Old age is a fact of life. I love to see and be around happy old folks. Some older citizens seem to refuse to slow down but enjoy their lives to the fullest. I sometimes see great-great-granny jogging with all the modern gears attached as if she was sixteen again. They go to the gym not to sit around and be spectators but to engage in physical fitness. You should see some pumping iron with not an ounce of muscle to be seen anywhere, just sagging foundations! Good for them!

Geriatric nursing to me is in so many ways like the flipside of pediatric nursing. We are dealing with the old who are sometimes young at heart. From time to time it breaks my heart to see folks who were once robust, independent, and mentally astute reduced to confused, forgetful, and childlike individuals. They just seem to be fading away! They sometimes ask the same questions a hundred times without any care in the world of getting an answer.

As one gets older, life takes on a whole lot of new challenges both for the aged themselves and their family members. Sooner or later the human machinery begins to show signs of wear and tear, and eventually we succumb to all sorts of illnesses and eventually death. Our geriatric patients are prone to falls, resulting in fractures that put great strains on their bodies. The pain they suffer is sometimes hard to deal with, and when some of them are medicated for pain control, the side effects of those medications sometimes leave them confused. It sometimes tugs at my heartstrings to see the aged attached to ventilators and other gadgets with poor quality of life. I ask myself, "Are we prolonging their lives or are we prolonging their deaths?" Prevention is the best cure, so my comrades-in-arms who choose that specialty try tirelessly to keep them safe and sound. They are in the forefront of infection control, nutrition, activity, and treatment of acute as well as long-term illnesses among the elderly.

People's culture, their value system, and their general outlook on life impacts to a greater or lesser extent the way they approach old age. Some embrace it willingly and go with the flow while others fight it! One ninety-nine-year-old woman who I had the pleasure of caring for in hospital after she was admitted for a fracture told me that she could hardly wait to get better so she could go home.

"Home? You mean a nursing home?" I asked.

"No sweetheart, my own home. Who wants to be in a nursing home with a bunch of old senile people? If you hang around those old folks too long, you will become old yourself. That place is not for me, sugar. No siree! And guess what? I live alone."

Just recently I cared for a 109-year-old *young* lady! Never dare call her old. She certainly had a sweet tooth. Not one tooth was to be seen anywhere, but just offer her some ice cream or cookies dipped in cold milk, and she was happy! I have had the privilege of also caring for many patients in their upper nineties and into their hundreds, and I deem those moments very special. They are like the finest most delicate china or crystals that you cannot afford to drop; they are to be handled with the utmost care.

The sad part of caring for them is that they have a limited amount of tomorrows. The friends from their childhood, pass away one by one, and I sometimes wonder if they think to themselves, "Who is next?" I am slowly learning and practicing the notion that I can and should live my best life today! Sickness, old age, and eventually death are just a step away from each of us, and every day we awake with the sun and see it set behind the western horizon should be a time of jubilation.

I love old people and old things. I love old movies in black and white and photo albums filled with black-and-white pictures crammed with beautiful memories. I sometimes wonder how folks in those bygone eras made those masterpieces, putting such vivid imagination into costumes and backgrounds and scenes. Those masterminds have long since passed on, but their legacies still remain to entertain, inspire, and help us appreciate the finer things of life. I believe that the most beautiful hymns we sing today, the cantatas and the anthems, were produced in the eighteenth and nineteenth centuries and that they are very hard to beat! The composers were in no rush to meet deadlines or to beat the clock. They had a lot of time on their hands to perfect their art and still leave us mystified and awed just by beholding and hearing those treasures. What can come close to George Handel's *Messiah*? We have to give credit where it's due.

I love writing poetry. I have composed more than sixty poems. Out of sheer inspiration I write! As a tribute to the golden agers and all that is related to being older, I dedicate this poem.

"Old Things"

Old things always have that special appeal.
If one observes closely one would feel
That special quality, that touch of class
That timelessness we dear not ignore or pass.
We view old art, antique, relics
That we sometimes get rid of or hide in our attics.

It's so nice to visit a museum
And see a broad spectrum
Of the way people lived in times past.
Their hard work and talent will last
So that generations yet unborn may
Come to cherish and their homage pay.

Oh the fine texture of old silk and tapestry,
Memories, mellowed with age, such luxury!
Old folks full of experience enough to speak volumes.
Old houses so private, so personal, one hardly fathoms
How and why they designed such constructions
Which escape all kinds of disasters and destructions.

We learn so much by reading old past history
Full of intrigue, suspense, and mystery.
Old stories, "Old wives' tales," fairy tales
The "Once upon a time in a far away place" never fails
To make us feel young and vibrant
Carefree, happy, and buoyant.

The thrill of seeing old folks staying together
For many years, through fair and foul weather.
Still the sweethearts as on the day they said
"I do," determined to stick it out to the very end...
Aging gracefully with gray hair and wrinkles
But their eyes never lose their twinkles.

Old photo albums with young and old faces,

Old love letters and postcards from faraway places,

Old songs that bring back memories of youth.

If you want to know the truth,

Those old songs give meaning to life and living

And are worth hearing and singing.

Check in great-grandma's cedar chest

You might still see her wedding dress

With the most delicate embroidery and lace

Fashioned with thoughtfulness and grace,

For who knows, a great-granddaughter somewhere,

May this very dress have the pleasure to wear!

Let us welcome the new but preserve the old.

They are worth a lot more than rarest gold.

Stick with your old pals, your old folks.

Don't see them as burdens or heavy yokes!

Keep your old pets, don't put them to sleep.

Let them sleep naturally; their memories are worth the keep.

When the workday is done

We all need some kind of fun.

Get your old slippers, slip in your old tired feet.

Go to your comfortable old chair, and take a seat.

Those dear old familiar "old stuff"

Will help you unwind and bring ease, more than enough!

Nurse Educators

There would be no nurses if someone had not gone before us and then been willing to train the next generation of healthcare providers. The success or failure of any nursing program depends to a great extent on the men and women who impart skills and instruction to students. I always had the desire to become a nurse, but until I was trained to be one, I was as ignorant of what nursing is as any layperson.

I have observed all through the course of my life that there are people who are endowed with special gifts that just seem to grow on them. I sometimes wonder if those talents are acquired or simply bestowed. Some educators who I have had made learning pleasurable, and I could not wait to put in practice what I was taught. I had confidence that what I was instructed to do was ethical, factual, and that if I followed those blueprints, my nursing future would be bright. They take upon themselves an awesome responsibility in teaching young "green" people how to become safe and caring nurses of the future. We do have safe and unsafe practices in nursing!

Those nurse educators, sister tutors, professors, or whatever name we choose to call them have got to be many steps ahead of their students in terms of theoretical as well as practical skills. They research, study, and go beyond the call of duty to help their students succeed.

In every area of nursing, there will always be nurse educators. They do their jobs behind the scenes, in the classrooms or in the clinical areas, for the love of the game so to speak and for the benefit of humanity. We owe them a ton of gratitude, respect, and accolades of praise.

Psychiatric Nurses

I sometimes ask this question, which is worse, a sick mind or a sick body? I guess that that is quite debatable, but until we come up with a reasonable answer, we are going to have mentally ill folks on our hands throughout our nursing career. My comrades-in-arms who choose the psychiatric specialty are a rare group of nurses who literally put themselves in harms way practically every day to care for those patients. They are constantly in the line of fire. Who knows what lurks in the mind of a mentally ill person? Those who have lost touch with reality, that's insanity at its worse.

There is a code that is used in the hospital where I work called "Code Gray," and whenever I hear that being blared over the intercom system, I hope and pray that my friends are safe because it signals that some patient or even visitor is being disruptive or out of control.

What causes people to become mentally ill? There are many and varied causes, and research is always ongoing. Mental illnesses sometimes run in families. They can also stem from environmental factors, abnormal chemicals in the brain, head injuries, birth defects, infections, and substance abuse. Psychological trauma, neglect, and poor self-esteem also play an important part. I observe that there is a very thin line between sanity and insanity and that a person's coping mechanism, support system, cultural upbringing, and the way he or she views himself or herself makes a world of difference to his or her mental well-being.

Our modern society has plunged us into so many stresses, anxiety, dread, and fear that it takes the love and grace of God to keep us sane. There is a very famous man by the name of Sigmund Freud who has left us with a wealth of information regarding mental illnesses. During my training I was simply fascinated with psychiatry. I learned that every behavior is motivated and is also meaningful. I never considered that area of nursing to be embraced as a specialty, but nonetheless, I lift my hat to those nurses who have made success stories in that field. They, in their own small way, every day help mentally ill patients cope, and many are able to return to society as well adjusted, functional individuals.

There are moments in everyone's lifetime, nurses are not exempt, when we experience some form of low point. Even the most optimistic, jolly person will feel blue, discouraged, and languid at some time in their life. "No one can look into the bright sunshine all the time, and continuous sunshine without rain causes a desert," I often heard my sage of a father say. During those moments, we have to remind ourselves that we are human and try to be gentle with ourselves. However, if those moments begin to turn into more that a passing phase, and if things begin to spin out of control, then we had better get some form of help. "A mind is a terrible thing to lose!"

Visiting Nurses/Home Care Nurses

Gone are the days when patients have the luxury of remaining hospitalized for many weeks be it for surgical procedures or medical/surgical health issues. They are sent home sometimes with basic instructions as to how to care for such things as catheters, drainage tubes, surgical skin staples and sutures, colostomies, and a whole host of gadgets which can at times seem very overwhelming to a layperson or even a nurse who becomes a patient. My comrades-in-arms, the visiting nurses come to the aid of such patients in the privacy and comfort of their own homes. "They bring the care home."

Those nurses go into homes and situations that are sometimes less than ideal, but their concern for the welfare of their patients gives them strength and courage to go, and they deliver. They care for the young as well as not so young. Some patients are sent home from hospitals to recuperate after some form of injury so visiting nurses deliver skilled nursing care to them until those patients are back on their feet. On the flipside are those patients who are chronically ill or terminally ill who need to have palliative care.

I believe that most folks would rather be cared for at home than be confined in a hospital or nursing home environment. It must be gratifying to know that nurses will be there for them when they need them, delivering care and compassion in one package. End-of-life care can be taxing for all concerned, be it family members or patients themselves. To die with dignity and no pain and to be surrounded by people they love best, must, I believe, comfort many a dying patient.

Visiting nurses provide counseling in nutrition, infusion therapy, wound care, and a host of skilled care. They aim to get patients as functional and as independent as much as possible. Family members are encouraged to be actively involved in all this planning and implementation. There is a lot of paperwork involved just as the nurses do in a hospital setting, but it's all in the game called modern nursing. Some nurses would rather do this type of service than be in a hospital. They just love being there for their patients at home.

Military and Uniformed Service Nurses

Wars have been waged since the earth was populated, and wars will still be fought until the close of time. People can sometimes act like selfish, wild beasts, dying for causes that sometimes seem so foolish and unnecessary to the rest of us. To such folks steeped in tradition, hate and the need for revenge and even death pushes them to war against other people and nations. Protection as well as defense are commonly the reasons why countries around the globe engage in such conflicts. I really look forward to the time when "I'm gonna lay down my sword and shield and study war no more" as that old spiritual song goes. I long for hope and tranquil living in heaven.

Casualties of all sorts result on the battlefields of the world. Our nurses in uniform and combat boots are *really* in the line of fire. There are many ranks in the armed forces that our nurses attain to, and there is no stopping them to become the best of the best. Can you believe that some of our comrades-in-arms are decorated officers with the rights and privileges of any other member in the field or wherever they chance to be? They deliver care to the wounded within their ranks as well as to civilians. They are a very disciplined group of people who have to think on their feet and make split-second decisions in sometimes less than ideal settings.

I visited the famous Arlington Cemetery some years ago, and as I stood overlooking a sea of white crosses, I thought of a song I heard many times before, "Where have all the soldiers gone? Gone to graveyards everyone." Those brave hearts gave their lives for their country to "let freedom ring." I look forward to the time when there will be no need for my services as a healthcare professional. I will be put out of business; so will the doctors, paramedics, pharmacists, ambulance drivers, and the members of the armed forces. The tumult of wars will cease. I will sing lustily yet another inspirational song, "There will be peace in the valley for me some day."

It all sounds exciting and gives me a feeling of euphoria to be out on the battlefield defending a cause as well as saving lives. During the Crimean War Florence Nightingale and Mary Seacole left a legacy that is so honorable and noteworthy. Even as I write, there are nurses on the battlefields of Iraq and Afghanistan risking their lives. Isn't life, and nursing in particular, one great adventure! Some of us enter this noble profession after changing a career or two only to find ourselves changing specialties time and time again. We embrace bold undertakings with the willingness to get involved and take uncertain risks, even at the expense of our lives. Some of our armed forces' nurses remain on the reserve list only to spring into action when their undaunted services are needed. One hundred gun salute to you all!

Administrative Nurses

Somebody has to keep the ship afloat. Someone has to be the general, the boss, and the overall administrator. That person should be able to make rock-solid, sensible decisions for the good of the institution using his or her heart as well as his or her head. Nursing is no exception to this rule. Education, preparation, and leadership skills are all plusses that administrators need.

The titles given to the administrative staff differ from one country to another. Some are called directors, matrons, nurse coordinators, nurse managers, and sisters. Some categories are even distinguished by the uniforms they wear. The color of their belts, their headgear, or some type of pin affixed to their uniform tells who they are. Gone are the days when some administrative nursing personnel don uniforms and caps. They wear well-tailored suits and dresses or lab coats.

I have observed over the years of my career in my country and in North America that the administrators who are willing to listen to their staff, who show genuine interest in their employees, who are there for their staff through thick and thin, who are willing to roll up their sleeves and give a much needed hand when the need arises, most times, get very good dividends. When nurses are conscious of the fact that their nurse manager is looking out for their best interest, then the job, the pressure, the lack of coffee breaks, and the long hours seem more tolerable. I also observe that those of us who are reminded of how lucky we are to have a job or are constantly told to "do your job because it's what you are paid to do" are less likely to perform at our peak, use up more sick time, are more disgruntled, and, as humans, are prone to do far less than our best.

Those who are in charge of us need to be reminded that we are basically sailing in the same vessel and that we can be like the Queen Mary or the Titanic depending on the captain and the environment in which we navigate. Unless we own the institution we are all employees! Diplomacy, tact, and human kindness go a long way. The power to hire and fire bestowed on some of the folks in administration is sometimes taken to extremes. Granted, some employees will test those persons in authority to the limit if they are given free run.

Disciplinary measures are sometimes needed to keep the ship afloat. One bad mango sometimes spoils the whole bunch. Even though most of us love mangoes, we cannot afford to lose the whole bunch! But "encouragement does sweeten labor."

The schedules, the vacation time, the paycheck, the yearly evaluation of each staff member, the problem solving, and the overall planning have to be done by those who choose that line of nursing specialty. Nursing is revolutionary. We are constantly changing our approach to the methods and ways of doing things, but at the same time, we have to adhere to the highest standard of care.

To My Other Comrades-In-Arms

As I remarked before, nursing is revolutionary. I hope to mention as many specialties as I possibly can. I am no authority or spokesperson for any nurse, but my intent is to celebrate our achievements as a cooperate body. A few years ago a good many of today's specialties never existed. Now we are just about everywhere, and we are here to stay and make our presence and expertise felt and known. There is no stopping us, no siree! Take for example forensic nurses. Who would have believed that we could be right there on the crime scene collecting evidence alongside law enforcement officers!

We have nurse practitioners with the license and the privilege of making diagnoses and prognoses and writing prescriptions! I simply love them. They make life a little easier for me. Then there are nurse anesthetists. They administer both local and general anesthetic to patients and are not only capable of putting those patients to sleep but are just as competent in waking them up! Of course, God is the greatest anesthetist. He puts us to sleep at night, or anytime we choose to sleep, and wakes us up without using any chemical means. He does that even in the natural world. The birds, the animals, even the trees of the forest get some downtime, and as the sun makes an appearance, all nature sings and comes alive once again. No one can beat that. He is, indeed, an awesome God!

Public health nurses have been practicing in that field for a good many decades. I remember as a kid that I chose not to like them very much. I associated them with injections and bad tasting green colored medication that made me want to puke! They would "inflict" my arm with needles bearing vaccinations or inoculations. Sometimes my poor body would be roasting with fever as a result of those vaccinations. In those days I couldn't even pronounce that big word properly so I called it vaxcination. I can now look back and thank them for helping me fight all sorts of childhood illnesses that now threaten millions around the world to extinction. Infant mortality is still with us, and those nurses are at the forefront in the prevention of those diseases, which, indeed, can be prevented or even eradicated. They are involved in so many aspects of community life, and it's really amazing that even though they are most times few in number they are able to cover so much ground.

AIDS/HIV nurse specialists focus on the person who is affected by that deadly disease, and they are not too concerned about how and why those folks are affected. The reasons are not always trivial, but the hope and encouragement and their physical presence with those patients takes a little edge off the dread of those killers. There is still no cure for AIDS/HIV, but medications seem to be giving those affected a fighting chance, and I have personally seen survivors of many years. Some patients I know even volunteer to try out new drugs and have made success stories for themselves. The drugs, plus their will to survive, make a world of difference.

Research is still ongoing, and precaution is still taken by those courageous nurses along with the rest of us. We cannot afford to let down our guard because blood and body fluids are still the mode of transmission.

Ambulatory care nurses save many a patient the need to be admitted to hospitals for relatively everyday procedures. Gone are the days when patients are admitted for cataract surgeries, colonoscopies, gastroscopies, intravenous antibiotics, blood transfusions, and some types of chemotherapy. Some of those procedure are done right there in the Ambulatory Care Unit or are preformed in the operating room, and patients are returned to the Ambulatory Care Unit. That area can be quite hectic, and those nurses have got to make sure that current laboratory works, EKG, X-rays, and a whole host of pre-operative must-haves are on those patients' charts before they are ushered into the operating room. It is fast-paced unit because some of those procedures need very little recovery time before they are sent back to the Ambulatory Care Unit. Sometimes patients are seen in that department who are later admitted to the hospital following surgery.

I have a very soft spot somewhere in the region of the right side of my heart for children. I am not quite sure what difference that area of my heart makes, but that spot is reserved for them! I sometimes become quite uncomfortable when I see them with chronic illnesses that limit their lives, so I avoid caring for sick kids in a clinical area. Camp nurses are there especially during school breaks to take care of those precious young persons so that they are made to feel special while spending time at summer camp and in the great outdoors. I imagine that those times spent with other children must be the highlight of their vacation.

Some of my comrades-in-arms work in correctional facilities. Their patients are people who are in the custody of the state for some type of wrongdoing. People become sick whether they are free or incarcerated, and they need to be cared for by nurses. Those nurses working in that specialty are really in the line of fire, but there are some nurses who do not mind one bit being there. "Someone has to do it, so why not I?" they often say. Some of those patients are seen on an out-patient basis for routine tests and procedures while others need round-the-clock care, and that's exactly what they get without nurses getting personal or judgmental. They are truly professionals.

Wound care nurses also embrace another specialty area, that of ostomy care. Some patients have surgeries and for some reason or another end up having a colostomy or ileostomy. I imagine the emotional trauma most patients feel even if those ostomies are temporary and reversible or even worse if they are permanent. Ostomy care nurses work along with those patients and their families to educate, support, and help them adjust to their new challenges. The first hint of readiness to accept or even care for the ostomy I believe is when patients take a look at the bag attached to their side, muster the courage to touch it, and then begin to ask relevant questions. Those nurses try to custom-make supplies for each patient because one size does not always fit all. I guess that those patients' daily prayer is to accept the things they cannot change.

We have nurses in the areas of legal consultation, pain management, infection control, case management, toxicology, organ transplant, hemodialysis, substance abuse, developmental disabilities, dermatology, occupational health and rehabilitation, and documentation specialists, just to name a few areas! Each specialty is just as important as the other. I guess we all like to brag about what we love to do best, but at the end of each shift the most important thing that each of us needs to reflect on is, did I do a good day's job? If the nurse can answer in the affirmative, then that nurse will be able to sleep comfortably when he or she glides between silk sheets and places his or her head on the pillow! Why silk? It's a good investment; it's better than cotton; it lasts a long time; and it does a body good!

Chapter Twenty

We Are Not Alone

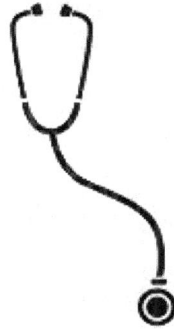

Nurses cannot and could not function in isolation. Even though we are practitioners in our own right, we need other categories of workers to complement us. Hospitals, nursing homes, clinics, sanitariums, and other places where people go for medical attention are manned by throngs of competent workers. The oft repeated quotation, "A chain is as strong as its weakest link," rings true for these institutions.

Nurses and doctors should, in my opinion, be partners in the care of patients. Sometimes that opinion seems lost in the shuffle. I would love to have a doctor volunteer to work a twelve-hour shift in the role of a nurse; I wonder what his or her reaction would be when the shift was finally over. Would a change of behavior occur because some form of learning took place?

My coworkers, nursing aides or nursing assistants, are among my favorite people on the job. I was trained to do what they do, and I can do it just as well, but their function is different from mine, although it is just as important. Just give me a few good nursing assistants and I know my patients are safe and comfortable. Most of them have a keen sense of observation. On many occasions they have called me to check on a patient because that patient "does not look so good," and trust me, their concerns are usually valid. When they give a bed bath, patients not only look clean but they have a baby-fresh clean! They are licensed to practice in their scope, and most of them love what they do and get great satisfaction in caring for those who cannot take care of themselves.

Patients need food. That is a basic need of every human being. They need to have meals planned and served to meet their individual health issues. The dietitians, nurses, and doctors work closely to ensure that the right types of foods are given in an attractive, timely, nutritious, and palatable fashion. I will never forget for a moment the hundreds of folks who sweat behind those hot stoves and ovens to deliver three or more square meals to our patients every day. That, I believe, is an enormous task and responsibility. I was told back in nursing school that cold food should be served cold and hot food should be served hot, and the dietary department tries hard to live up to that expectation.

It sometimes breaks my heart to see how much food is wasted by some patients and the constant complaints about the food. I can't help but think of the thousands of individuals who go to bed hungry or who are always preoccupied with where their next meal will be coming from for themselves and their families. I sometimes chuckle to myself when I see starving homeless individuals come into the hospital. They are given clean clothes, and they demand triple servings of food, but they still complain about how the food tastes like dog food, although they eat almost everything that is served to them. I wonder what qualifies them to make that comparison! In spite of all that, we need our dietary staff. They really deliver even though they will never be able to satisfy everyone's palate. I once heard a preacher say, "Some folks have food but no appetite while others have good appetite but no food. We should be very happy and grateful when we have both at our disposal!" That statement is so simple but so true.

Literally tons of linen are used daily in hospitals and nursing homes. Patients have to be kept clean and dry and comfortable. No one can ignore a wet patient and sleep comfortably at the end of a shift unless that person had his or her conscience seared with a hot iron. The smell, the shivers, and the discomfort of those patients, especially those who cannot express their needs, will come back to haunt you. Our housekeepers work side by side with the nursing staff to provide adequate clean sheets and towels so that our patients are happy. Housekeeping goes a bit farther than just providing linens. They collect the garbage, which by the way, might even add up to tons daily as well. They keep the surroundings clean. Disinfectants, toiletries, and a safe environment is key to us all.

Maintenance and biomedical engineering personnel provide us with so many indispensable things. We use all sorts of medical equipment and devices in caring for our patients. They undoubtedly break down at times. Take for example, medical oxygen and suctioning tools. We dare not have them broken when we need them! All of the monitors, pumps, alarms, and beds must be in good working condition at all times. We could not work without them. Then, of course, for those of us who would rather die than walk up six flights of stairs, there will always be the need for elevators. Our maintenance staff keeps us warm in the winter and comfortable in the hot summer months. They also keep the fire alarms and extinguishers in mint condition.

A lot of times we help people get better by chemical means. We do so by administering prescription and non-prescription drugs, which are calculated and dispensed by knowledgeable pharmacists. New drugs are manufactured and introduced to healthcare facilities so frequently that we nurses often have very little time to research those medications. I can, with ease and comfort, call up any of the pharmacists with whom I work and ask and receive information regarding any unfamiliar new medication or even how to calculate their dosages. Our pharmacists are in my corner when I need them.

Most times before a patient's diagnosis is confirmed, the patient's blood chemistries and blood counts and blood gasses help us determine the course of action needed to best treat that patient. Our laboratory staff is the group of people who I admire and depend on every day. If a patient has critical laboratory values, those technicians will make sure that the nurses or doctors are duly informed so that the necessary actions can be taken. In most every emergency, blood is drawn and sent to the laboratory stat, and before long, the results are ascertained, and we can then and there have some idea of how to proceed

They have to be very sure that the right names are placed on the right tubes of blood. If they goof up, heaven help us; that would call for some bloodletting on their part! Can you imagine getting a test result that is not yours? Some favorable ones that give false hope and some not so good ones that cause stress and sleepless nights? They are so careful to affix the name of the patient to the patient's blood tubes at the patient's bedside so as to avoid any problems! Accurate labeling is not only confined to blood but indeed everything we take from patients: cultures, tissues, body parts, body fluids, you name it, the right name has to be placed on them.

Some of our phlebotomists obtain blood specimens from veins that do not seem to exist. I often chuckle to myself when they arrive early in the morning with their cheery little voice and smile. At the same time they are armed with a patient's most dreaded weapon, a needle, and then they say, "Good morning Mrs. X, my name is ... and I am here to take a little blood from you. Just hold still while I tie the tourniquet and put the needle right here."

But the patient's response is not so pleasant, "You again, vampire? You took a quart of blood from me just yesterday, and you are back for more today? You folks must be selling my blood for money! As soon as those nurses put blood in me, you come and take it right back." Some of those patients bluntly refuse, while others just go with the flow and say, "My doctor told you to draw more blood today, didn't he?"

Let's talk a little bit more about labeling. When a baby is delivered the baby and its mother and father are tagged immediately with the correct information. Can you imagine being switched at birth? The fact of the matter is it does occur every once in a while. My siblings and I were all delivered at home by competent midwives in attendance, but ever so often when we were little and got on each other's last nerve, we would wonder if we were really related.

On the flipside of birth is death. The bodies of our dearly departed patients had better have the right names affixed, the right address, and the right family members notified. It would be an absolute fiasco if the person being eulogized is not the intended one. So it is very important that we be properly label when we are hatched and when we are dispatched!

Some other very important coworkers with who we nurses interact are the radiology, ultrasound, cardiology and EEG (Electroencephalogram), and EKG (Electrocardiogram) technicians. Illnesses, some acute while others are chronic will be with us as long as time lasts. Those department and clinical areas are always busy and unpredictable. Who knows when someone will be brought in with a fracture, chest pain, heart attack, or obstruction to some part of their anatomy who needs urgent testing by those highly skilled and efficient technicians. We sometimes take for granted the care we give to our patients, and we sometimes do so by sheer reflex action because of our experience and routine. I am glad that those folks are available when I need them in our quest to save lives.

Our modern society has been increased with knowledge to render higher standards of healthcare. People most times do not die from illnesses that plagued folks some sixty years ago, but our behavior has declined sharply. Some people have become fierce, rude, uncouth, and downright lawless. We need the security personnel to keep us safe. Most all hospitals have codes that are activated in response to emergencies. One of them in my institution is "Code Gray." Security personnel usually respond immediately to the area where the actual or potential disturbance is occurring. I feel much safer when they are around. If needs be, they will solicit the help of others to bring calm and safety to our hospitals and clinics. I sometimes refer to them as our own Homeland Security!

There is another group of coworkers with whom I have a great rapport, our unit secretaries or ward clerks as they are sometimes called. With such fine workers around, the stress seems more bearable. They answer the phones, make sure our much-needed supplies are available, communicate with just about every category of worker in the hospital, and are, most times, our best advocates!

They alert us as to what changes a doctor might have made regarding a patient's treatment and what needs to be done right away because they are right there. Let's face it, nurses cannot always be at the nurses station, so those unit secretaries process the doctors' orders in a timely manner and relay the information for a smooth transition of care. It is every nurses' responsibility that we know what is going on with our patients. It's not the secretaries', but they play such an important role in helping us in such matters.

Then we have folks who work at the switchboard. When important information needs to be aired throughout the hospital, they get on the intercom system to let us know the latest news. They handle communication within and outside of the hospital. Then there are the folks who work in the medical records department, the billing department, payroll, admissions, respiratory therapy, and in-house transportation. A healthcare facility could never function at peak performance if those able workers were not there.

Some hospitals have chaplains assigned and they are most times available when needed. I can imagine the pain that they sometimes feel when they have to relay unpleasant news to family members or even be called to offer the last prayers for those whose time here on earth is almost expired. That's their calling, and they do it well.

Last but by no means least are the physiotherapists. I sometimes see them as miracle workers. People with all sorts of physical disabilities, be it from planned or unplanned traumas, improve their mobility and become independent once again thanks to the physiotherapists. This specialty is so broad, but whatever areas those folks choose, clients most times attest to great improvement and better function. I see patients with neurological problems, fractures, respiratory problems, joint pains, postoperative procedures get moving independently over a relatively short period of time.

Pain is and will always be a part of the human experience, but with the help of physiotherapy many a stiff, inflamed joint and aching muscle show great improvement. Fractures and joint degenerations are no respecters of persons. No matter how well those fractures, hip or knees, are repaired or replaced, without the involvement of the physiotherapists, those patients' recovery would be prolonged or next to impossible.

In my own small way, I have been showering compliments on the folks with whom I work as a nurse, and the team spirit in my hospital is one to be envied or emulated by others. I might have unwittingly omitted some, but in my heart everyone who works for the good of humans, just ordinary humankind, is special and very important. We seem to stay put and are not too eager to run off when the going gets tough or rough. Like a close-knit family we get on one another's nerve at times, but at the end of the shift we are family. I do not like to hear anyone put down the place that provides me with my bread and butter. In other words, don't speak ill of my hospital. Patriotism, loyalty, and gratitude go a long way in my book! I am happy, very happy to have a job; many people don't. I am sure glad we are all in this together because it would be sheer misery or hell doing it alone!

Chapter Twenty-One

What Lessons Has Nursing Taught Me?

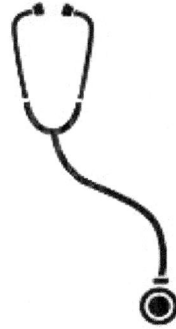

Nursing is sometimes difficult, but it is one of the most rewarding professions one could choose. I was told from day one that it's an art and a science. I will also add to that statement that it is love in action plus a lot of commonsense! We might not be sent off to do a tour of duty on the world's battlefields, brandish guns, or wear combat boots, but we are engaged in a war against diseases, some new and very frightening, ignorance, bigotry even in our ranks, and violence in the workplace. The famous Florence Nightingale and the Jamaican nurse Mary Seacole were involved in the Crimean War.

Love in action, eh! Nursing is sometimes based on tough love. Tough love is getting a patient up and out of bed the first or second day after surgery, sometimes under protest from that patient, but we nurses know that the patient will be the beneficiary a few days down the road. Tough love is literally putting ice on a patient or using a cooling blanket to bring down his elevated body temperature. Nursing is daily encountering blood and body fluids enough to make one sick if not handled properly. It's dealing with sweat, vomit, ulcers, maggots, and death—things that would make most folks puke. It's all about assisting in the introduction of a new life on planet earth and being there when one takes one's last breath and slips away into the cold embrace of death. It's research, it's cures, it's hope and great expectations. Nursing is pride, professional humble pride. It's fighting for a cause even if others think otherwise. It's going out on a limb to guide and to save our patients. I do not give my patients pity. Pity lasts for just a little while. I extend to them empathy and genuine love.

Nurses have to be vigilant and in some places, shifts are termed "duty." Day, afternoon, and night duty are done just like police officers on their beats! If we are found sleeping on duty, someone will rudely awaken us and then reprimand or even fire us. If for whatever reason we are not relieved after our prescribed duty or shift, and we walk out of that institution, then the charge of abandonment will be leveled on us, and we can kiss our jobs goodbye!

The first time I heard about the AIDS and HIV virus was in 1980 when I was living in Canada. My brother-in-law Milton heard the news item one morning and decided to pick my brain. "What is AIDS?" he asked me.

I didn't know what he was asking, so I gave him some definitions of the word "aides," which I thought were to assist, help, military assistant, grants, and so forth. The nerve of him to say to me in a very condescending tone of voice, "You call yourself a nurse and don't even know what that word means, shame, shame on you!"

I then asked him the million-dollar question, "What has nursing got to do with it?" That was when I realized that an old word had acquired a dreadful new meaning that has forever changed the way we live and even the way we view one another.

Just about everyone now knows about AIDS (Acquired Immune Deficiency Syndrome). Sadly enough after more than twenty years since it first came on the airwaves, a lot of ignorance and bigotry still surround this killer. Millions have succumbed, several millions are still living with it, and still countless numbers have no clue that they have this disease. During my training, some of today's diseases that could have been treated effectively with traditional antibiotics, rest, and proper diet have become resistant to even some very powerful broad-spectrum antibiotics, and this can be quite worrisome.

Nurses are exposed to all sorts of illnesses, and even when patients are quarantined or put on isolation for whatever reason, we still have to care for those folks, putting ourselves at risk. Sometimes just by sheer reflex action, we nurses rush in where angels would fear greatly to tread, shove our hands into just about everything to make sure our patients are safe. We seem to put our lives in the hands of latex and latex-free gloves, so we don a pair and are ready to do battle with all types of blood and body fluid. We sometimes get stuck with dirty needles and are bitten by patients. "Get bitten by patients?" Yes, you got that right, and please remember that human bites are potentially dangerous! We attend to people from every walk of life with many and varied motives and agendas, temperaments, and expectations. But we deliver! We are the rare breed of workers who see patients as real people, and not diagnoses, room or bed number, or diseases. Our creed is "my patients first."

It is said that God looks out for babies and fools. Most of us nurses do not fall into either category, but I really believe that God has a special place reserved for nurses. Let's face it, He is pretty capable of doing everything quite well all by Himself, but He also likes to delegate some type of responsibility to earthlings, so He chooses a special group of people who He knows He can trust to take care of the sick, and He calls them nurses. He seems to put a special shield around them, an armor of defense. I have never seen a nurse die on the job on his or her assigned shift!

We are oftentimes bombarded by staff shortages and verbal abuse by patients and their families. I have been around long enough to compare tabs. It appears that in some quarters, we have lost the high respect we once enjoyed. Did we contribute to its decline? In spite of the negative things that rear their ugly heads at times, we have within each of us the resilience, strength, and fortitude to survive and to make an important difference in the lives of our patients and their loved ones.

I have learned that our patients can become our greatest teachers and that we should be willing to be taught by them. After all, they know their bodies better than we do. Sometimes I meet patients who have very rare and unfamiliar diseases, which I have only seen in medical/surgical textbooks. So what do I do? I ask them to enlighten me. If patients question me about anything ranging from medication to treatment, I listen. One simple mistake could become somebody's grave! They might be telling me something that could very well make the difference between freedom and a maximum security prison, their lives and my license.

Nursing demands sacrifice and more sacrifice. I believe that one of the hardest things to do is to get out of a warm, cozy, comfortable bed in the dead of night and get into a cold car or wait at a freezing train station or subway stop. Sometimes nurses are the only creature breathing in the cold air on those nights. In one of Shakespeare's plays I did in high school, I remember this quotation, "Creatures of night love not nights like these." In wintertime the road conditions can become so treacherous that had it not been for the grace of God, we would have arrived at work via an ambulance! It's hard to tear ourselves away from our kids, sometimes sick kids to care for other people's sick kids and family members. I know what it means to have left my terminally ill father in a hospital bed to come back to care for other people's sick fathers and mothers. Sadly, the next time I saw my father was in a casket! On special occasions such as Christmas, birthdays, and Thanksgiving, when others are having a wonderful time, we have to catch a quick nap and be prepared to hit the road to watch others sleep. But we do it!

I have learned that some of us in the healthcare profession have very little compassion for folks who become patients for one reason or another. If we could just place ourselves on the other side or on the surface of those patients' beds, we would change our tune. We need to consider what it would be like to experience for ourselves or our loved ones a feeding tube, an IV going through our arm or neck or groin, a liter of fluid passing through our colon in the form of an enema, a colostomy bag hanging from our side, a bedpan squeezing our delicate buttocks, or a bout of nausea and vomiting following chemotherapy or surgery. If we were to look into the mirror and see a hairless scalp staring back at us after radiotherapy or chemotherapy, then those times and experiences would help to keep us human, humble, and compassionate. Unfortunately, some of us, if we experienced what our patients experience, would not be made better but bitter! We can become a bit haughty and heartless.

I have learned that regardless of what attitude I choose to adapt when I go to work, the shift will end! So I purposefully try to start off with a pleasant, positive one. It's not always easy, and even with my best intention, sometimes things happen that spoil my day. Someone rubs me the wrong way, or let me put it another way, if I choose to be rubbed the wrong way it might snowball into unpleasantness. How we choose to act or react to those unpleasant moments makes all the difference to the outcome of our shifts.

I have learned that the things we do to others can come back to bless or haunt us somewhere in the near or distant future. I have seen folks in positions of authority, women in particular, because let's face it, nurses are predominantly women, abuse those positions so badly that many a nurse has wept bitterly. "The female of the species are more deadly than the male!" I have also observed that time has a way of healing wounds. Those wounds sometimes get infected, and although they eventually heal, they often leave permanent scars! I have seen some of those oppressors suffer and die slowly and painfully. Those occurrences should not be deemed "good for you, you deserved that and more," but should serve as object lessons.

The road on which we nurses travel is not always paved with gold or other precious metals. The road is not without its ruts and potholes, but we can make the passage a little smoother for one another and for those who come behind us. On one occasion I tried to teach a nurse an important truth. I said to her, "We can catch more flies using honey than vinegar."

She said, "Oh no, you catch more using feces!" I substituted feces for the word she used!

I told her, "That might be so, but the process stinks!" She laughed.

Away from the halls of the hospital, the way we treat our patients and their loved ones also impacts us when we meet them in street clothes. A nurse told me that she had just finished the evening shift and was heading home in a not too safe place to walk in broad daylight let alone in the dead of night when she felt afraid and alone.

As she walked she, every once in a while, saw two individuals behind her, so she walked a little faster. After a while she saw only one person and she wondered, what next? Finally, she reached her bus stop and began to catch her breath when the person who was following her made his presence known. This was what he said to her.

"Nurse, many months ago I was shot, and I almost died. I was admitted to your ward and you took good care of me. When I was discharged, you even gave me the bus fare to get home. That man who was following you was going to hurt you, but I took care of him. I will stay with you until your bus gets here. Nothing bad is going to happen to you as long as I am around. I followed you almost every night since I was discharged, but you did not know. I was just trying to pay you back for all that you did for me."

She had mixed emotions. Did he harm or even kill someone to save her? What if she had not been kind to him in the past when she had a chance? How should she respond to this person who elected to be her hero? Chances are, he would have taken care of her had she not been compassionate to him. We as nurses need to be very careful how we treat the people God loves as dearly as He loves each of us. Remember, "Inhumanity of man to man is the greatest sin" and "A good name is rather to be chosen than great riches."

I have come to realize that we are blessed with the gift of healing. There is no substitute for skilled, experienced nurses. It is acquired by being at the bedside, the stretcher, the crib and giving hands-on, honest to goodness, unselfish tender loving care and doing for the patient that which he or she cannot do for himself or herself. Most times we do not get the credit for what we do, but we play our part well. That's the crowning beauty and glory of being a registered professional nurse. I believe that we nurses need to be one hundred percent committed to our calling or we become a liability rather than an asset.

I am a patient advocate. I think we have embraced some misplaced priorities, and we need to get back to basic common sense nursing. How would Florence Nightingale and Mary Seacole react if they visited a hospital in North America in 2013? Undoubtedly they would be extremely impressed with the great strides nursing has made. They might say, "You've come a long way, baby." But they might not be able to finish a twelve-hour shift and come out alive! The "lady with the lamp" might be mesmerized or completely awed if she had the pleasure of holding a flashlight or seeing how electricity works instead of carrying around a lamp to check on her patients!

The advancements in the medical field might be too much for them to handle. They might even die from a heart attack! But I do not believe they would appreciate the limited time spent with our patients and the ceaseless paperwork that nurses do today. Paperwork is fast becoming extinct. Staring into a computer screen for ceaseless hours is now the way to go! I believe and try to live this maxim that my parents drilled into my consciousness from childhood, "To thy own self be true!" In the meantime I have to adhere to the notion that "not written, not done!" We need to get real and give back to the nursing profession the honored place it once enjoyed in our towns, communities, and in the world. We have the power to change the world, a little at a time, one shift at a time, but the change must begin with us.

Nursing has transformed me into a believer. A believer in or of what? A believer in miracles. I have seen the awe of life and death, the first and last breaths, and I still stand amazed. That's nothing short of a miracle. I believe that nurses, doctors, and everyone who has a hand in the restoration or healing of the human machinery is an instrument whom God uses to accomplish His purposes. I believe that it is not farfetched to give of ourselves unselfishly every day for the benefit of our patients and be left depleted or deficient. I believe in letting people know what I stand for and what I will never put up with under any circumstance!

I believe in the cause of nursing. I will live for it, but I will not die for it! This has been my theme since I first donned my blue and white uniform, and it will continue to be so until I clock out for the last time into retirement! A very good Man, a very long time ago, laid down His life for His friends, including me, but I am not willing to do so for anyone, unnecessarily, at this point in my career. A dead nurse is of importance only to the undertakers!

I believe that when we as nurses become so puffed up with our importance and status as professionals we should ask ourselves this very important question, "Ten years from now will I be remembered by anyone in the institution that I am now employed?" There is no vacuum in nature! That goes for our self-importance. "Do you remember that tall beautiful nurse who used to work on ... floor? Her name was Milicent."

"Milicent who? I have no idea who you are talking about. She must have been dead and gone a long time before my time but who cares?" How dare they forget me! But that is the reality of life. Nurses come and go.

I believe that we need to get back to the times when our patients and doctors respected us enough to call us by our given names in the workplace. After all, do we not address them as Doctor Brown, Black, Purple as the case might be? I believe that when a doctor yells out, "Milicent!" in the hallway, I should be able to say, "Yes, Tom, what's up?" or as Bugs Bunny says, "What's up, doc?" I am not allowed to call my patients on a first name basis so why should they feel free to call me Milicent? My patients and I are not pals. I am their nurse. Granted, there are individuals who I have grown to love dearly within the confines of the hospital. I think of them as being a part of my family. That's okay. Feel free to call me by nice terms of endearment, within limits of course!

I believe we have made some very significant strides in nursing in terms of prevention, technology, and achievements. I sometimes look back to the beginning of my career and laugh out loud. Sometimes it's difficult to look into the past and to face the future. I remember caring for patients who had relatively simple everyday procedures done and we were ever so careful of how we turned and positioned them. Patients who had a laminectomy or some other types of surgery were confined to bed for several hours post operatively. No wonder some of them developed all sorts of complications afterwards! Nowadays, many surgeries and surgical procedures are being done via the ambulatory surgical areas and doctors' offices, and patients are discharged from there with instructions related to their care at home. They are sent home with all sorts of gadgets in place. To my amazement and awe, I now see patients who have had spinal surgery getting out of bed within a few hours and being discharged the next day. What a difference a few years make!

Instead of randomly opening up a patient for exploratory surgery, we now have all sorts of diagnostic tests to pinpoint what the problem is. Take for example, MRIs, CT scans, and test related to nuclear medicine.

Those tests most times are all-inclusive as to what is happening to a patient and the course of action to be taken by the doctors. These days, the end product of some major surgeries is just a few bandages to the patient's abdomen. During my time of training those tests were slowly emerging, but now they are the norm.

I firmly believe that our bodies are fearfully and wonderfully made. It seems almost comical to realize that countless numbers of individuals we meet every day in the street are walking around with a lot of missing body parts! They have missing teeth, prostate glands, uteruses, kidneys, lungs, appendixes, spleens, pancreases, legs, tonsils, you name it, but they are still able to function well. Years ago, chances are if those vital parts were removed then those patients would have been removed from the land of the living!

We are successfully separating conjoined twins, doing open-heart surgeries, transplant surgeries, laser surgeries, and all kinds of noteworthy neurological procedures that are being fine-tuned and getting better every day. We are using high tech procedures to allow women to have eight children in one shot! "The more the merrier!" We are rivaling rabbits and pigs. Eight, that's more than enough! One woman's uterus stretching to accommodate eight babies, that's incredible, that's king size! I believe that research in so many fields will one day, maybe not in my lifetime, enable us to find the key to eradicate diseases such as cancer, sickle cell anemia, diabetes, and a whole host of others that have become more prevalent over the past few years.

We have been searching for the fountain of youth for as long as time itself, and many people have taken steps to dig those wells or find them gushing forth like streams in a desert land. Some folks have become cosmetic surgery junkies, and some doctors are there just willing and waiting to assist them to discover how, when, and where those springs and fountains are. We now have facelifts, tummy tucks, liposuction, breast reduction and enhancement, gastric bypass, skin peeling, and a whole host of plastic surgeries to make us look and feel better about ourselves! Sometimes we don't quite get what we bargain for and our savings in Citibank or on Wall Street take wings. I once saw someone with huge scars around her ear line and brow line. Her ears seemed quite deformed to say the least. I asked her if she had ever had any injury or burn to her ears. She informed me that she had a facelift done some years ago. Her skin was stretched taut, and it seemed as if she had a perpetual grin on her face. The scars looked like tribal markings!

Some plastic surgeons, however, have a love affair with their scalpels and know exactly how to wield them to create masterpieces. When they are finished and those bandages are removed from the targeted spots, the end results are out of this world, and I mean, some of those folks look "out of this world." Some folks really get their money's worth. They experience beauty and endless delight and are thrilled.

Some folks try very hard to lose weight, and I really believe that it's a constant uphill struggle for them. How they packed on those extra pounds is not the all-consuming issue. How to get them off is more important. I believe that we as nurses have the means by which we can teach our patients better alternatives to some of the foods they consume that directly contribute to weight gain. Gastric bypass has become quite popular. The risks are still great, but some folks swear by them. We can try to develop a love affair with fruits and vegetables, nuts, whole grains, and liters of plain old-fashioned, honest to goodness water. An investment in a comfortable pair of sneakers or a membership at a gym with the determination to sweat and sweat some more is sometimes all it takes to lose and keep off weight. But it is never by any stretch of the imagination easy to do.

I have read several books written by Dr. M. Scott Peck. One of my favorites is *The Road Less Traveled.*

The first sentence in that book, consisting of three words, got my attention: "Life is difficult." Dr. Peck doesn't claim that during our lifetime everything will be fabulous. If we were given such beautiful promises of a life without pain, stress, accidents, struggles, setbacks, sweat, and broken dreams and promises then those monsters would creep up stealthily on us when we least expected them, and we would be miserable. When we are cognizant of the fact that life is, indeed, difficult then we can gear ourselves to meet those challenges hurled at us and plan accordingly. Addiction or any other vice with which we are plagued is hard to kick, but we can eventually get those monkeys off our backs with determination, faith in God, and hard work. We cannot just wish them away, we have to work at them.

Nursing has taught me that things change over the years in our personal and interpersonal lives. We do not dress the same way we did twenty years ago; we do not necessarily look the same way or think the same way either. Amid the ceaseless changes and counterchanges that assail us, who we really are remains unchanged. Our love for our chosen profession, the care of the most important person in the hospital bed or crib or incubator, the person on the operating room table, in the recovery room, or in the clinic does not change. That love mellows with age.

Experience, time, care, and the tenacity to hang in there and be the best and to impart our knowledge and skill to the next generation of nurses as we make a triumphant exit into retirement deepens and broadens our love for all that's called nursing. Some people just have the unlimited capacity for giving love with very little expectation for getting anything in return. That's the glory of nursing! We sometimes find hope and give hope in the midst of the storm, on the battlefields, and at the bedside of our patients. But it is worth the trip and some of us would not have it any other way!

Only very recently a patient reprimanded me for not telling him that I would be off for two days! "Am I not entitled to have a few days for myself?" I asked him.

"No, no, not when I am here as your patient! And by the way, how many patients have you taken care of on a one-on-one basis during your career?"

"Can you count stars in the night sky?" I asked him.

His warm smile made me realize that somewhere along the way I must have been doing something good.

I have "come of age" in nursing and have seen many seasons come and go, and I have learned that the most important place for any nurse to be is exactly where he or she is today. Just being here at this moment in one's life does not happen by chance. We can become the best we possibly can. When we give of ourselves unselfishly without demanding or expecting anything in return, people take note of that fact. We sometimes beat ourselves up wondering if we are good enough nurses and if we need to change. Most patients whom we have had the pleasure of caring for over the years, love us just the way we are and would not want us any other way. I have learned that each nurse has that moment of self-discovery when she or he stops and shouts out loud, "Wow! I did it for my patient, and I have no regret in doing it because deep in my heart I knew that it was the right thing to do." Whatever that *it* was, that nurse did it! That's his or her Kodak moment, picture perfect!

Chapter Twenty-Two

Now, May I Make Some Positive Suggestions, Nurses?

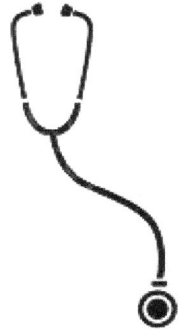

Nurses, my comrades-in-arms, these are no patronizing, condescending, lecturing, or "who does she think she is?" type of suggestions. No way! Every once in a while, we all need some word of hope, encouragement, and affirmation or a gentle reminder to face the long dreary hours during our shifts. Especially to our recent nurse graduates and those who have not yet received any or many battle scars, I will try to show you the ropes in my own small way. I am now descending the mountain and facing the western sun with its long shadows behind me, but I will face it with integrity and fidelity. I am speaking gently to myself as well, so here we go.

When the need arises, sacrifice a few small moments out of your busy shift, pull up a chair, and sit by your patient's bedside. Only when the need arises! Those extra minutes won't hurt. You can still hold your patient's hand without donning a pair of gloves. There is no substitute for a non-threatening human touch. We are dealing with human beings and not diagnoses. We have embarked upon a time when everything seems to be taken out of context. Gone are the days when we could kid around with our patients or anybody for that matter, within limits of course. We now have to be careful, very careful how we address them lest we be sued for all sorts of harassment. Discretion cannot be overstated.

Avoid like the plague or the swine flu any personal confrontation with our patients. Even if we win, the victory will be short-lived and not very sweet. There will be patients who will deliberately make life miserable and will even try to tarnish our reputation and threaten our licenses. It is said that no one should contend with anyone who has nothing to lose! Never should we waste our beauty sleep on them or torment ourselves over them. They will eventually be discharged, and chances are, we will never see them again. If it gets so unbearable, trade them off for ten other patients! Believe me, there will be other nurses who will be willing and able to take care of them.

Never be afraid or intimidated to question any doctors' orders, written, telephoned, or otherwise. That is our bill of rights, and those queries might make all the difference between sleeping in a jail cell or being in the land of the free and the home of the brave.

We need to have a strong hand but a gentle touch. No "iron hands in silk gloves!" I once saw a sign posted over the entrance of a labor and delivery room, "Not by force, just by skill."

The tongue can be a very dangerous tool. If it gets loose at an inappropriate time, it can cause untold damage. It's very hard to tame. Sometimes in order to keep it in check, even for a brief moment, we have to bite it! Bite it for peace sake. No way am I suggesting that you should roll over and play dead when a situation calls for taking a firm stand when dealing with what is morally right or wrong. Believe me, there are certain things that are not worth sweating or arguing about. Time and age have taught me that truth. We can never win over some patients or their families or even some coworkers, no matter how hard we try. Life is too short to be spent on debates and strife.

Take a well-earned vacation or a few days off before you get burned out and miserable. Do you have sick time? Of course! It is good to have a "mental health day" every once in a while. Don't abuse sick time, and don't lie about the reason off such as saying, "My mother just died, and I have to catch the next aircraft out," when your mom is sitting right beside you and is as strong as an ox going nowhere close to any grave! A word to the wise is sufficient!

Keep abreast with current trends in nursing. If you don't, chances are you will be left behind, and it's hard to catch up.

Use humor as a safety valve when the pressure of work assails you from every quarter. If I were to take everything my patients have dished to me over the years, I would have been placed in a psychiatric hospital with four-point restraints. I try to see the funny side of things.

Guard your license viciously day and night. Trust no one with it! When you lose it for whatever reason, it's very hard to have it reinstated.

Never put in writing anything that can be misunderstood, misinterpreted, or questioned. This can land you in jail, and remember, lawyers are a very expensive breed of professionals. Don't commit the sin of omission! Chart what is necessary in the interest of time, good judgment, and commonsense. Unwritten information can come back to haunt you in a court of law. Stay focused on what's important.

Encourage and be supportive of student nurses and new graduates. Deal gently with them because, trust me, you are going to need them when you become old, demented, and not knowing the difference between your grandkids and a broomstick standing in the corner or that you were once a nurse! Nurses are people too. They have a very long memory span, and they might remind you of a thing or two if you were mean to them when they needed you. I remember the kindnesses showed to me in my "growing up" years in nursing by those who were there before me, and I have always endeavored to reciprocate and encourage others to do the same for young nurses.

Ask for help when you think or know you need it. I have observed that some nurses do not hesitate to delegate some of their responsibilities to other nurses at the drop of a hat, while others try to be independent. Regardless of how long you have been a nurse, you will never know it all. Let me rephrase that statement. There are some nurses who act as if they know it all, but check their performance, and it leaves a bitter taste in your mouth. They are all talk and no action, and they make sure that the right people hear them at the right time! Have you ever met any of those folks?

"Big winds blow loudest in empty caves," and "Empty barrels make the most noise." Some of those folks happen to get some real lucky breaks when the time is ripe for them! They know all the policies and procedures but do not know how to implement them. They would rather walk on the other side of the unit just to avoid checking on a piece of equipment or pump that is alarming or call on someone else to fix it!

Save your back by practicing good body mechanics, and call for help to lift or pull up patients. I started out with good body mechanics, and I will end with it. This might sound so matter-of-fact, and we should know that, but how many times do you perform tasks that cause you harm that might have been prevented? Back surgery is very expensive, so is physiotherapy. As for the pain, that's another story. We all know that back injuries can sometimes result in pain or leave you crippled and handicapped. Take care of your precious back.

Pamper your feet. They carry your tired body all day long even though most people take them for granted. Sometimes to get your attention they ache, cramp, and get numb. Give them a good soak and massage at home or pay professionals to handle those toes with respect and tender loving care. Don't worry about the expense; they are worth it! Those feet were originally designed to last a lifetime, and you can't afford to wear out those soles the way you wear out your sneakers, boots, and shoes.

Never make promises to your patients that you know you cannot keep, and don't give them false hopes. Many of us are not licensed to write prescriptions and make diagnoses, but we are experienced and observant enough to know when a patient is not going to make it out alive from a hospital bed. Sometimes family members come to you expecting you to give them assurance that their loved one will get better soon. I usually refer them to the attending doctors or residents. Let them deal with the prognosis. I don't hold out hope in obvious hopeless situations, neither do I have the last say.

Be very careful, very careful what you say in the presence of your patients. Remember that the sense of hearing is the last to go. When you believe that they are comatose and are not hearing you, think again! They might eventually wake up and take legal action against you and hold you accountable for character assassination.

You have to sometimes set limits for your patient's behavior. They don't necessarily have to love you, but they should have some measure of respect for you. Nursing is an essential service, but it is not to be viewed as some domestic servant's position. We are nurses, not servants. One day a patient's family member called me "girl" and demanded a cup of coffee, not for the patient but for herself. I informed her that I did not wear a bib, carry a tray, or take tips waiting tables! To this day, I do not think I was rude. I told her the truth with an air of dignity and professionalism.

Never be too quick to give too much advice. Make positive suggestions to your coworkers as well as to your patients. I learned this truth very early in life. By asking, "What do you think?" sometimes solves many a problem. When we make positive suggestions and give hints, then the person wishing to get answers might just see the light and make their own decisions without much prompting. If they did not get what they bargained for, they will not be able to lay any blame on you.

When the going gets tough, very tough, remember that all this shall pass, just like kidney stones! One day a student nurse observed me taking part in a code (for cardiac arrest) on my unit. When it was all over, she asked me how I remained so calm during the whole ordeal while she was stressed to the max even though she was not involved. I gently informed her that it might get worse before it got any better for her. I, however, reassured her that with time, she might be able to do great and that a calm, unruffled attitude to an emergent situation helps everyone cope better and more effectively.

Let's take good care of ourselves and one another. Sick nurses cannot take care of sick people.

Pray at the start of the shift, in the middle of it, and at the end of it, and pray some more! I usually sing a song silently when I am stressed. I do not "sing like the nightingales, so I sing like the gales in the night!" A song is such a beautiful thing that goes straight to the heart!

Try as much as possible not to ask your patients too many personal and private questions. Trust me I have learned!

"Is this your husband?"

"No, he is my son!"

"Is this your wife?"

"No, she is my daughter!"

"How is your mom doing? I took care of her on several occasions."

"My mom died twenty years ago!"

"How old is your baby now?"

"What baby? I have never been pregnant in my entire life!"

"The last time I saw you, you looked very pregnant to me. Sorry, my mistake."

"Are you losing weight?"

"NO! I have put on twenty pounds in the past three months!"

Some folks just like being "well upholstered," so don't even think of suggesting Weight Watchers or Jenny Craig to them! They will kill you. A doctor with whom I have worked for years usually tells his not-so-thin patients to try to look like me before they are discharged from the hospital. I try to keep the weight off. They would take one look at me and ask him if he is crazy. One patient told him, "The day you look like her, that's the day I will look like her!"

Don't be afraid to cry. There is nothing like honest, sincere tears. I have been in situations where I am caught up in my patients' concerns and predicament. Those moments can become real tearjerkers, and patients and their families sense your sincerity, and although the "I understand how you feel," is not uttered, the message is received and appreciated. Empathy and understanding go a long way. Even the Son of God was not afraid to cry publicly. He wept!

I observe that nurses seem to be the world's fastest eaters. We just chop and swallow. Who has time to settle down and have a decent lunch or coffee break? We sometimes unconsciously act as if we are at the waterholes in the African jungle buying time to get a quick drink before we are chased away for whatever reason then later on we lie down to chew our cuds! Every once in a while make a conscious effort to give your stomach the respect it deserves by sitting and chewing like the rest of the population. You are worth it. Take a few moments of luxury!

Never try to be perfect. I have seen some "very perfect" nurses fall on their own swords or be escorted from their place of employment by security. Never be too quick to report to your supervisors every little thing that your coworkers do for crying out loud! Some love to write up their counterparts for everything. Some just love to have a conference call with the administrative staff! We shouldn't condone mediocrity, incompetence, or downright negligence, but "discretion is the better part of valor." Remember, we all work and live in glass houses, so we had better be very, very careful how we throw stones at one another! The nurse who has never made an error, forgotten to do a procedure for whatever reason, omitted an important document, or shown up late, can cast the first stone! We all goof up at one time or another.

Retire at your pinnacle. Leave gracefully while you can still walk out independently and not be carried out via a stretcher or pushed out in a wheelchair. Leave with a bang, a clear conscience, and a good reputation. Don't hang around until people begin to pity you or are too willing to pull up a chair for you so you won't fall and break some important body part. After you have worked hard for what you have, spend some time enjoying it. You don't have to flaunt it, neither should you express any remorse for it. When you leave, don't look back. A wise man once said, "Don't outlive your money! And select a doctor your own age so you can grow old together." Solid advice I would say. What do you think?

Do something that will change someone's life for the better and will add a fresh appeal.

We are always at the forefront of teaching our patients the importance of keeping in shape, thus reducing the risk of developing illnesses down the road. But very few of us sacrifice the time to exercise. We have the prescription, so why can't we find the time to fill it! Long hours on the job, school, children, and a host of other "important things" surface when getting on the treadmill or walking is mentioned. We need to live long enough to enjoy our retirement, which comes a day closer every shift. Park the car and walk. Every once in a while drive into the countryside and see Mother Nature's handiwork. Enjoy the good life before arthritis takes up permanent residence in your joints! Keep your minds active. Do crossword puzzles or write poetry or a book. Trust me, those are not always easy things to do, but they are worth it!

"Life and Living"
Are there fountains of youth?
I'll tell you nothing but the truth,
I do not really know,
But if there were, I would certainly go
And stick around forever
Do I want to get old? No never!

We will all become old
That's the way it is, we are told
But we don't have to hasten its arrival.
This might sound trivial,
But we can remain young at heart
For as long as we want.

God wants us to have good health
Coupled with prosperity and wealth,
Peace of mind, a guilt-free conscience
Beautiful smiles and cheerful countenance,
Gratitude for all His love and care
And the willingness to serve others and share.

Good health doesn't come by easy
No excuse for being too busy!
It's good to take daily walks in the sunlight
Breathing deeply and filling our lungs, that's right!
We need to exercise as well as rest
If we want to be looking our very best.

We need water, no substitute is good enough.
Drink to your heart's content, that's good stuff!
It will keep your skin soft and blemish-free,
Rid our bodies of toxins, relieve constipation, you'll see!
Curb appetite and help in weight loss,
Cheaper than going to the gym, it's free of cost!

We all want to feel and look good.
Fruits, nuts, vegetables, and wholesome food
Can help accomplish that and so much more.
Exercise keeps us fit, gives us more energy than before.
It helps relieve stress, anxiety, and tension,
And guess what? It even controls hypertension!

Start a journal. Rekindle the flames of letter writing. The mail carrier used to be a welcome person each time a delivery was made, not necessarily bills but letters from friends and relations. Telephones, computers, and a whole host of modern gadgets have robbed us of the joys of communicating via the post office. Old love letters and old postcards are still treasured by the ones who have seen many mango seasons come and go such as I. Sentimental as well as passionate is what I sometimes describe the people who prefer to express themselves in writing. Read a good book. Elizabeth Barrett Browning wrote, "No man can be called friendless when he has God and the companionship of good books."

Chapter Twenty-Three

Positive Suggestions to My Patients

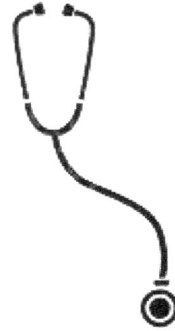

It is so hilarious at times to note how quickly our status or titles change in just a short space of time. We get out of our cars, off the bus or train walking and talking as we usually do, then in a split second we enter a doctor's office, a dentist's office, a chiropractor's office, clinic, or hospital, and suddenly we become *patients*! Most times we are there for just routine physicals or only to let our dentists know that our teeth are in good shape and working condition, but our title changes until we leave those buildings and step outside, hopefully with a clean bill of health. When my dentist refers to me as her patient, I sometimes ask myself, is she speaking to me or about me? Funny, isn't it? I bet you never thought about it that way before!

Believe it or not, when you get to the hospital or clinic or even your doctor's office, your freedom is restricted, even if it is for a short time. You will be told what to do! Nurses will tell you to take off your clothes, get on a scale, get into bed, submit a specimen, and even take out your dentures if necessary. We sometimes take away your valuables and put them away in safekeeping for you. A great number of us hate to strip down in front of strangers. Thank goodness for clothes! Of course, nurses do not overly expose you, but they like it when you cooperate for your own good! Who wants to be labeled non-compliant or uncooperative? Just tell yourself that all this will pass just like kidney stones and is intended to help you get better, eventually!

When you become a patient for whatever reason, planned or as an emergency, pray to God to send you a good nurse because she or he will protect you from all the other not so good healthcare professionals. Next to God, no one will take better care of you than a good nurse! At the same time, don't take her or him for granted. They have warm blood running through their veins; they are humans, and some humans don't forget or forgive easily. We are trained to act in a professional manner at all times. Show me a person who has never gotten mad at some point in his life, and I will tell you that you are dealing with someone who is in a state of rigor mortis! Long dreary nights, full bladders, uncomfortable shoes, constant "nurse I need this, I need that!" soon get to even the most disciplined human. Be careful, we can snap under pressure!

Keep a list of your medications handy to be given to your doctor or nurse. Know if you have any known allergies and your vaccination status.

Don't be intimidated by doctors, nurses, or other healthcare professionals. Remember, those folks are living, breathing human beings like yourself and every once in a while they get sick too. Be sure you understand your bill of rights when you go to a hospital. Read the small print, and don't be afraid to request a second opinion. Remember, "the big print *giveth* and the small print *taketh* away!" Only give consent for those procedures that you feel comfortable with after you have been educated about the risks and benefits. Do your homework and ask pertinent questions. Avoid asking questions just for the fun of it. Try not to bombard your nurses and doctors with too much irrelevant farfetched stuff that you happen to see on television, read on the Internet, and just want to pick their brains about. They have more important things to do, including taking care of you, the most important person on this side of the mattress!

Know as much as possible about your medical history, the types of medical problems you have, and the surgeries you have undergone in your lifetime. That information might be able to expedite the proper diagnoses and determine the appropriate plan of care.

Get involved in your own care and that of your family members. Many times I see family members come to visit their loved ones and then come to the nurses station stating that their loved one needs a glass of water when they could get it themselves and give it to their loved one. Put some lotion on Mommy's feet and arms, comb her hair, fluff up her pillow, and show her how much you care. The aides as well as the nurses are employed to take care of your mommy's needs, but I strongly believe that relatives and friends who come to visit can contribute a little of their time to care as well. There is no substitute for the personal touch of loved ones and kinfolks.

If you have pain, let someone know and request relief. A few pain relievers won't transform you into a junkie during your hospitalization. I do not handle pain very well, so I make every effort to keep my patients relatively pain free. The reality of it all is this, not everybody will be a hundred percent pain free in his or her lifetime, but we can try to take the edge off the discomfort.

Do not expect your nurse to take away your independence. She will not be bathing you, combing your hair, brushing your teeth, and do what your barber or beautician does for you when you can, indeed, do those things yourself. That is a luxury she cannot afford. Nursing is doing for you that which you cannot do for yourself. If she does all of that good stuff for you, before long you will become an invalid, and if or when you do return home, believe me, your wife or husband will not put up with you if you pull those pointless acts on him or her. He or she will give you the boot! We are not callus or mean-spirited nurses. When the need arises, we will surely pamper and give you all the TLC you really *need*, not want, but only until you regain your independence. You will never win, but you stand to gain full recovery as a functional human being! Paradoxical, isn't it?

Advance directives are here to stay so be sure you make your wishes known regarding treatment or lack of treatment you desire. Failing to put those wishes in writing might be the moment of truth you never bargained for. Those documents won't speed up your entry into the casket, but a well-informed and well-educated patient is a joy forever! We nurses simply adore you!

I do not subscribe to the notion that patients are always right. *No, you are not always right!* No one is always right a hundred percent of the time. But you have a right to be heard and seen and to be treated with the utmost respect and dignity. Don't abuse that right!

Never trust a doctor who is afraid to tell you, "I don't know the answer to what's ailing you, but I will be more than willing to refer you to someone else who I *know* and *trust.*"

I once saw a billboard that I found so very amusing. A layperson had a stethoscope on a doctor's back. The sign said, "Examine your doctor before he examines you." How true! Treat your doctor as an equal associate and partner. You should have mutual respect for each other. If that very important ingredient is missing, do a bit of "doctor shopping," and believe me, there are many out there who are willing to see you, sometimes even without an appointment!

Think twice about seeing a doctor whose waiting area is very crowded with sick folks, and in a relatively short period of time, they are all treated and sent home! He is a doctor and not a magician for Pete's sake! He will not give you the attention you deserve or pay for. If patients are there only to pick up an already written prescription, then that's a different matter, but each patient deserves personalized, undivided attention and time with his or her physician.

Turn off your cell phone when you go see your doctor. He or she will be turned off by the distraction of a ringing phone.

Chapter Twenty-Four

Forward Unto the Future

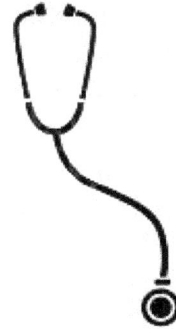

Some dreams are so real they could be easily confused with reality. My dream of becoming a registered nurse as a five year old stayed with me every waking moment of my life. I could not shake off that feeling no matter how hard I tried. Dreams are useless unless implemented so I did all that was needed to actualize it. Some folks live out their dreams while others bury them. If I had not pursued my goal it would be as if the firmament was stripped of its innumerable galaxies. "Impossible dreams" do come true, but sometimes we have "to be willing to march into hell for a heavenly cause." I have been celebrating the days, weeks, months, and years since I cast my lot with the millions of nurses living and those who have passed on, and I stand tall and proud.

Nursing is the totality of reality. It can be filled with love, history, mystery, suspense, and cliffhangers—it might even be in stiff competition with the most watched and loved soap operas. I sometimes reflect on the stories I read as a kid. They most times began with "once upon a time" and climaxed with "and they live happily ever after." Those happy endings I have lived, indeed. The truth is this, our patients need us and most times adore us. We have come to the kingdom for such a time as now or then. No one knows for sure what the future holds for the nursing profession.

The whole world seems to be spinning out of control. At times I feel like saying, "Stop this universe, I want to hop off!" There is, however, a Person in charge who holds the future in the hollow of His hand. He is always on call and He never calls in sick. He is involved in every emergency. He takes care of our equipment, our supplies, our staffing, our salary, and our retirement funds. He does not need unions to bargain or negotiate for us. He has the authority to hire and fire as He chooses, but He gives us second chances and His evaluation of our performance is always just and fair. He is the epitome of what an excellent Administrator should be. Nurses, our future is very secure if we trust Him with our todays and tomorrows. We have His assurance of having red-letter days. *He is God!*

"So This Is Nursing!"

I saw myself "there" as a nurse at age five.

I did everything to keep that dream alive.

I studied hard, was focused, and was eventually accepted

Into a school, old but highly respected.

I am part of a great healthcare profession

To prevent and cure diseases, that's our intention.
I have the ability to make life miserable and sad,
But I choose to make my patients' happy and glad.

I have seen the birth of a child, the awe of a new life.
I have seen death, pain, grief, suffering, and strife.
I have seen miracles, I believe in them because I know there's a God.
I've seen trust, imparted hope through good times and bad.

I have stood by the bedside of the sick and dying.
I've seen anger, pleading, acceptance, sighing.
I've gone beyond the confines of the hospital and bedside
To the funeral home and the graveside.

Do I have regrets for choosing this profession?
No! It's a struggle, a challenge, but a lot of compensation.
Would I trade it for another job? A thousand times no!
I'll always love and stick to this "evil" I know.

We invite you to view the complete
selection of titles we publish at:

www.TEACHServices.com

Scan with your mobile
device to go directly
to our website.

Please write or email us your praises, reactions, or
thoughts about this or any other book we publish at:

TEACH Services, Inc.
PUBLISHING
www.TEACHServices.com • (800) 367-1844

P.O. Box 954
Ringgold, GA 30736

info@TEACHServices.com

TEACH Services, Inc., titles may be purchased in bulk for
educational, business, fund-raising, or sales promotional use.
For information, please e-mail:

BulkSales@TEACHServices.com

Finally, if you are interested in seeing
your own book in print, please contact us at

publishing@TEACHServices.com

We would be happy to review your manuscript for free.

www.ingramcontent.com/pod-product-compliance
Lightning Source LLC
Chambersburg PA
CBHW080334270326
41927CB00014B/3218